THE WOMAN'S
WORKOUT BOOK

THE WOMAN'S WORKOUT BOOK

Anna Selby and Alan Herdman

the
apple
press

ISBN 1 8507 60772

This book was designed and produced by The Paul
Press Ltd, 22 Bruton Street, London W1X 7DA

Editorial: Annemarie Whittle, Robert Cathcart
Designer: Bill Mason
Art assistant: Sue Brinkhurst
Artists: Sheilagh Noble, Coral Mula,
Iona McGlashan
Photography: Don Wood

Art Director: Stephen McCurdy
Editorial Director: Jeremy Harwood
Publishing Director: Nigel Perryman

Typeset by Wordsmiths, Street, Somerset
Origination by London Direct Colour Offset Ltd
Printed in Great Britain by
Purnell Book Production Ltd.
Paulton, Bristol

Contents

Foreword

What associations come into your mind when you think of exercise programs, exercise studios and gymnasiums? If you allow yourself to be guided by the media, you will almost always associate them with the finished product – the sleek, supple, bright-eyed and clear-skinned woman, or the slim-hipped, wide-shouldered man, with good muscle definition and an impossible skin tan. In real life, of course, this is simply not the case, so, right from the start, throw away these false images.

First of all, do not be disillusioned if you do not fit into the mould promoted by the media. Second, take a long, hard, honest look at yourselves and decide not only what needs to be changed, but, even more importantly, what actually can be altered. Fitness and well-being are one and the same; they should be promoted and cultivated on an individual level.

So start by stripping off and standing face on to a mirror. Are your shoulders drooped and rounded forward, do you have a waistline or a roll of flab and what about your stomach? Turn sideways. Is your head jutting forward and are the shoulders and upper back curving forward? Does your lower back curve in, making your stomach and butt stick out?

Where do you go from here? Still standing sideways, gently tighten your buttock muscles and pull in your stomach. Lengthen your spine, pull back your shoulders –you should feel your head being pulled gently up, away from your body. See the difference and, much more imporantly, the possibilities. By improving your posture –

or just by standing up straight – you are already using muscles that have been dormant. Through the right kind of exercise and just a little self-discipline, this can become your natural, comfortable way of standing and moving.

So much for the externals. What about the internals? Obviously, standing up straight and freeing the torso is going to make breathing easier. But do you breathe enough? Think about this carefully. Since any form of exercise uses up a lot of oxygen, it is important to build up the cardiovascular system, which delivers oxygen to the muscles. This is an extremely important part of any fitness program. You must consider your life-style as well. Do you over-eat, drink too much and smoke, for instance? Do you eat an excessive amount of junk food? Do you make do with the minimum amount of sleep and allow yourself to become tense and irritable? All these factors play their part when it comes to deciding what you should do to achieve the maximum degree of fitness and physical and mental well-being.

Take all these points into consideration before starting on the actual routines and programs given in this book and you should be able to recognize and release the full potential of your individual physique. Bear in mind, too, that there is no age limit – exercise is not just something for the young. It is something that should continue throughout life, chaging slowly as you grow older to suit the inevitable ageing processes. Whatever your age, it is never too late to start!

Why weights?

Why do you want to shape up? Are you tired of looking at yourself in the mirror? Have you found that you can't quite squeeze into your favorite dress or pair of jeans? Are you frightened of being the ugly duckling beside the pool or on the beach? Whichever your reason, you have got as far as picking up this book. What you have to decide now is not only whether the workout programs it gives will work, but why you should follow them in preference to the countless other exercise options open to you.

Let's start with a few basics. First and foremost, you should understand that there is simply no wrong reason for deciding to get in shape; what is wrong is that people all too often approach the subject with quite the wrong attitude. If, for instance, you see your body as something you can starve, pummel and bully into shape, you could not be more wrong. This approach may work in the short term – you could look good for your entire summer holiday, say – but, unless you are ruthlessly determined, you will simply find that you can't keep the discipline up for all that long. It's so easy to relax and let go, to stop your exercises and for bad habits to reassert themselves. The result – you are back to the same old you.

If this pattern is all too familiar, now is the time to change it for good. Decide here and now to get yourself in shape – and to stay that way. The exercise programs that follow will stretch and tone you, conditioning your body until you reach a peak of vitality. And the bonuses this brings will spill over into every other area of your life.

There's sound scientific logic to back these statements. Each time you exercise, a hormone called Norepinephrine is released inside your body. This hormone is nicknamed the "kick" hormone because this is precisely what it does; it gives you a natural high that makes you more alert and increases your general sense of well-being. Conversely, exercise of the right kind helps you to unwind, relax and sleep better.

You'll notice that the word "exercise" has just been qualified – and for good reason. Just as there are "right" kinds of exercise, there are wrong ones, in both individual and general terms. To understand this better, let's take a brief look at the whole fitness phenomenon before looking in detail at the programs in this book.

The 1980s will go down in history as the fitness decade. All over the world, people of all races and all ages came to realize that their general level of fitness affected every aspect of their health and their determination to do something about this led to the fitness boom, typified by the interest in jogging and aerobics. Unfortunately, though, such extreme forms of exercising have proved too

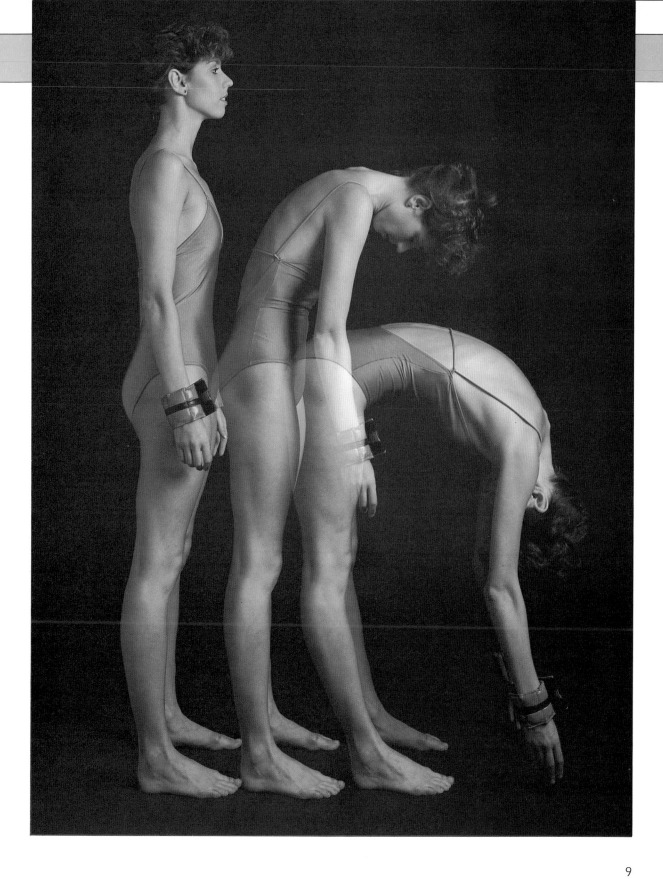

strenuous for people who had led sedentary lives for months, if not years. The repercussions were inevitable – jarred backs and knees and even undue heart strain.

For this reason, the approach to fitness and health has been modified. People are now much more informed about both of these vital subjects and tend to follow a more holistic approach when it comes to looking after their bodies. So they think carefully about diet, are wary of stress, appreciate the importance of rest and relaxation and are aware of the risks of smoking, alcohol and drugs. And they take a gentler approach toward exercise as well.

EXERCISING ALTERNATIVES

When you decide to start exercising, the key question you should ask at the start is "what is the most suitable form of exercise for me and my lifestyle?" There is only one answer – a regular, gentle program that builds up as your own physical capacity increases. This applies regardless of whether you are exercising on your own at home, or at a keep-fit or dance class. Going to a such a class once or twice a week is invaluable, provided that your instructor is observant and well-trained. He or she will correct you and help you to discover your own postural bad habits – unfortunately, we all have these – and help you to learn how to extend your body's strength and suppleness.

It's a good idea to combine other forms of exercise with your program, too. Swimming, for instance, is one of the best all-round forms of exercise, and any outdoor sport is good for you, provided that you recognize your limits and build up your involvement in it gradually. The one thing you must not do is overstrain your body, as otherwise you run the risk of injury.

WHY USE WEIGHTS?

Though all these activities can be of great benefit, they will tend to put the emphasize on one part of the body, whether it is your heart or your biceps. For whole body toning, or for work on a specific problem area, a more concentrated effort is required.

This is where the weights described in this book can be so useful. If you work through the exercises carefully, you will not only end up generally fitter; you will also be able to firm up flabby arms, or slim down thighs. Don't expect the weights to work miracles, however. There is no such thing as a magic answer to your body's problems and, just as with any other exercise system, body toning with weights requires an effort. But, given that effort and sufficient time, you can transform your shape.

WILL I END UP MUSCLE-BOUND?

Many people assume that by using weights they will end up looking like Mr. Universe! Understandably, this makes them anxious – and this is where the weights on which the exercise programs in this book really differ from the normal variety. In conventional weight training, the body literally builds up to take the strain of the really heavy weights involved, and, by the very nature of the movement involved, the muscles have to bunch up with the effort, so becoming typically muscle bound.

HOW DO THESE WEIGHTS WORK?

When you use the weights specified in this book, you are working almost all of the time with a weight of 2lbs per limb and occasionally with a maximum of 4lbs. This means that the muscles do not have to turn in on themselves with the strain. In fact, the reverse is true – throughout the book, you are constantly reminded of the need to stretch out your limbs to their limits, so extending the muscular line. This constant emphasis on muscle elongation certainly gives them strength, but this is the dancer's strength of a long, toned, controlled line. This is one of the reasons why these weights have always been so popular with dancers. There is no jerky lifting involved.

YOUR OWN PROGRAM

You can use weights as the basis of your fitness program, concentrating on the thirty minute routine, adding a dance calls or swim as you prefer. Or you can use them as a toning tonic or simply to help out any area of your body which you think needs extra work.

The choice is yours. But, whichever way you decide to use the weights, they can be your key to a sculpted, transformed you.

Getting down to basics

For any exercise program to work, you need to follow each part of it correctly. Although this may seem to be stating the obvious, most exercise programs are not followed accurately. Apart from people "cheating" on their exercises, most exercise books only show the detailed movements sketchily. Even in formal exercise classes, all too many teachers fail to explain enough to their pupils, or to provide sufficient correction when this is required.

The danger of exercising incorrectly is twofold. First of all, the exercises will not work as well as they should, and second, you also run the risk of hurting yourself. This is why this book sets out the basic principles of posture and movement right from the start, and returns to them in all the subsequent exercises.

If you are starting from scratch – or almost from scratch – the first thing to remember is that you should never push yourself beyond your limits; you can work hard without straining your body beyond its capacity. Begin by trying all of the exercises without weights, and then build up gradually according to the star codes (Each exercise is marked with one or more stars, the more stars there are, the more difficult the exercise). The exercises in this book are all based on 2 pound weights.

The second principle is to learn how to use your body properly. The complex interconnections between arms, neck, back, legs, stomach and indeed every part of your body should be understood if you are to get the best out of exercise. So, let's start at the top!

HEAD AND NECK

Something which is often forgotten is that your neck is an integral part of your spine, so you should always keep it long and in alignment. In practical terms, this means that you should not allow your chin to jut out or tilt upwards. Keep it down, so that you are looking straight ahead. It is important to concentrate on this as it also helps to release tension in the neck which is a very common problem.

Remember that your head weighs a considerable amount. Many of the exercises, such as the one shown opposite, utilize this fact to a great advantage. Here, the position of the head draws out the whole length of the spine and straightens it. You can see how the head should be held upright on a strong, straight neck for good posture. Achieving this is one of the most important of your exercise program's priorities.

SHOULDERS

Like the neck, the shoulders are a common seat of tension. An all-too-frequent tendency is to hunch them up – so drop them down! If you do draw your shoulders up, make a mental note to check their position as you exercise. If they are tense, circle them, or circle the head.

ARMS

All arm movements start from the middle of the back in the shoulder blades – not from the shoulders themselves. Tension and distortion are usually caused in the neck and shoulders by moving the arms wrongly. To learn how the correct movement feels, take your left arm behind your back, so that the back of the hand rests on your right shoulder blade. Now slowly lift your right arm up and out from the side, feeling the movement in the back in the back and keeping the shoulder well down. Try the same movement, lifting the arm up in front of you, and then try it on the other side. Bsides the movement in the back, the arms should feel comparatively weightless.

In any of the exercises that involve holding out the arms at the sides, they should stay in line with the body or slightly in front of it. Don't let them stray behind.

BACK

It is vital that you always keep your back straight. Many women have S-shaped backs, and stand with both their bottoms and stomachs protruding. This is not only bad for the spine, but also looks unattractive. Hold in your stomach muscles and lengthen and straighten the line of your spine, so that you can almost feel the air between each vertebra. You can find the correct line for your back by looking at the picture opposite and following the exercises on pages 30-31.

STOMACH

You should always hold in your stomach lightly but firmly as a matter of course, as the muscles here are central to

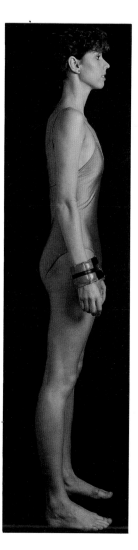

balance and posture. But though this rule also applies during exercise, take care not to put too much strain on your stomach muscles. If your stomach muscles bulge during an exercise, it means you are pushing them too hard, too soon: you may also be putting undue pressure on your back as well. If it is an exercise against weights, try it without the weights until you become stronger.

Do not curve your back when doing stomach exercises – concentrate on maintaining your posture throughout. Breathing is also important. The muscles should be working hardest as you breathe out; if you do otherwise, stomach muscles are more likely to bulge.

THE CONTRACTION

The contraction is a movement which is an integral part of many of the exercises in this book and it is vital to understand it properly. It includes a pelvic tilt – which means pushing the hips slightly forward so that there is no curve in the small of the back and the spine is lengthened out – but it actually involves much more than this one area.

The movement starts as you breathe out by pulling the stomach muscles up and back – feel as if you are pressing the navel against the spine. As you do so, tilt the pelvis forward so that the small of the back rounds gently and the buttock muscles tighten. The combined effect of these two movements should open up the whole pelvic area so that the thigh muscles "wrap around" – feel as if the inner thigh is trying to face front! In the rest of the body, there should be no tension, and the chest and shoulders should be soft and open.

LEGS AND BUTTOCKS

It is a common problem for many women that the thigh and buttock muscles are not used to their fullest extent. So when you are doing the exercises for this part of the body, make sure you can really feel the effort in the right place. If you don't feel it where you should, correct your whole body position until you do. It is very important to really stretch out the leg, elongating the muscles to their fullest extent as you do so. If the exercise calls for pulled up muscles, make sure you feel the movement right trough the leg into the buttocks.

A further very important point in leg/buttock exercises is that they require a firm effort to be made in the stomach. Because your legs are heavy to lift – even without weights – this can mean a great deal of effort is needed in the stomach, too. If at any time you feel the strain of a movement going into the back instead, you should stop as you are not yet strong enough for the exercise. In this case, try it without weights or, if this is still too much, choose one with a lower star rating.

POSITIONS AND TURN-OUT

In ballet, there are a number of basic positions for the legs and feet, but in this book we use only three. The first, parallel, means exactly what it says. The feet and knees face straight to the front. Always remember that the knees should be straight, the muscles above them pulled up.

First position has the heels together, the toes pointing outward in a V-shape. The movement starts, though, not in the feet but at the hips. The legs turn out from the hip sockets. Never try to turn the feet further than the legs can turn in the hip sockets or you will upset your whole posture. The knees should always be directly in line with the feet. If your feet are turned out more than the knees, you will find that the knees roll inward.

Second position has the feet apart – about 18 inches – and turned out as in the first position. Again, the legs turn from the hip sockets and the knees should be directly above the feet.

BREATHING

The most important thing to remember about your breathing is that the effort of any movement works on the out-breath. So, if you are doing a plié, breathe out as you go down; or, if you are lifting your leg, breathe out with the lift. If you breathe out with the effort of a movement it will be easier to pull up in the stomach and push the navel back toward the spine.

In the stamina sequence in the Basic Routine, concentrate on the out-breath, as this will keep the breathing regular. Never hold your breath with the concentration of trying to do an exercise properly as this tends to build up tension – and this, above all, is something you should try to avoid whenever possible.

Pilates exercise

Whatever your exercise program, you need to be involved in it mentally as well as physically. If you start thinking of it as a chore, it will become one – and be skimped, or given up, in consequence. For this reason, it can pay you to combine home exercise with regular workouts at an exercise studio. Simply working out with others can be a great mental tonic, while a sympathetic instructor can help you to iron out faults and problems.

What you need to be able to do is to distinguish a good exercise class from a bad one. While a lot obviously depends on the personality and degree of involvement of the instructor, there are also key basic ideas to take into account. What this means is finding the exercise philosophy that suits you and your body – there's no point in trying to follow an exercise program you don't enjoy simply because it's supposedly good for you.

THE PILATES METHOD

Walk into a typical Pilates-based studio and you should be able to sense the atmosphere immediately. You will probably see four or five people gently rotating their legs in long stirrup-type instruments, squeezing large cubes of foam between their tighs, or laying flat on their backs, slowly gliding up and down the plié machine, a kind of trolley attached to springs – all to the soothing background of classical music. There is no sense of rush, no feeling of competition against the other exercisers or yourself, no merely mechanical exercise apparatus. Here, you exercise body and mind, since advocates of the Pilates method aim to achieve a truly total sense of mental and physical well-being.

BIRTH OF THE METHOD

The Pilates system originated around 80 years ago in Germany, when a frail child called Joseph Pilates took up body building to increase his strength. The program he devised was so successful that, by the age of 14, he was posing for anatomical drawings!

But the great breakthrough came about almost by chance, as one of the only good things to come out of World War I. Pilates had moved to England, where, as a German national, he was interned on the outbreak of war. It was during the war that the true method was born.

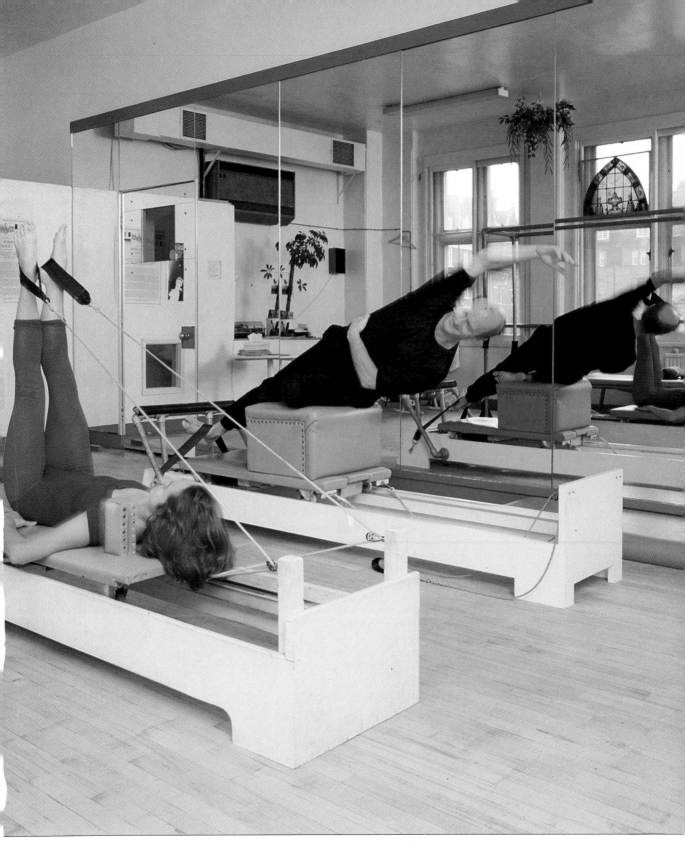

Pilates called his new system "muscle contrology". In it, he aimed to bring about the complete co-ordination of body, mind and spirit through working with – not on, or against – the body's muscles. The ideal was a totally harmonized and balanced human being.

After the war, Pilates returned to Germany. There, his methods won quick acceptance in the dance world, an association which has continued to the present day. Dancers immediately recognized the unique part "contrology" could play in limbering, strengthening, toning and stretching their bodies, safe from the risk of physical damage. Then, in 1924, he and his wife Clara moved to New York, where he opened his now world famous studio, devoted to the principles he had developed.

Dancers were the first to flock to the new studio. George Balanchine, founder of the New York City Ballet, said, for instance: "To live on this earth it helps to have a healthy body. Here is a way. The Pilates Way. It is wonderful for your body, wonderful for your muscles – particularly those of the stomach and back. I have used the Pilates method – I still do. My dancers use it and it works."

Along with Balanchine, Jerome Robbins, Martha Graham, Hanya Holm and Ted Shawn were all among the method's keenest devotees. And Ruth St. Denis, the "first lady" of American dance, said: "Not only is the body rejuvenated, but the mental and spiritual refreshment is beyond calculation."

PILATES TODAY

Where dancers led, sportsmen, actors and the public followed. The method spread across the United States and back to Europe. Often, there has been so much adaptation that the exercises bear little resemblance to the originals, but some teachers still remain loyal to the original Pilates principles.

I am such a teacher. I studied the Pilates method in New York and have taught it in the United States and Britain. On first sight, my bright, airy studio looks rather like an obstacle course! It contains about 10 different pieces of equipment placed at various levels and angles, all featuring a number of curious attachments – springs, pulleys, bars, handles and weights. They are based on the machines in the Pilates studio in New York.

As well as the machines, you will also find conventional weights, which are used after a work-out on the machines, when the body has been warmed and stretched. Dumbbells are used for what is termed "definition" – they are especially good for flabby arms and flat chests – while the ankle weights are used mainly for "spot reductions" on thighs and bottom.

The exercises themselves are deceptively easy. Some are simple limbering and toning up exercises, done on the floor, which you can do at home between classes. Others use pulleys and weights as a force for the body to work against – what is known as dynamic tension. They are slow, strenuous and many of them are similar to the kind of movements dancers do at the barre. For example, at the beginning of each class, you do leg stretches, or pliés, just as you would at the start of a formal ballet class. The only difference is that here you do them lying flat on your back, aided by springs. This means that you can really concentrate on stretching, strengthening and controlling specific muscles. It also means that the exercises are much easier to do.

In the Pilates method, you will find that lying on the back and working against resistance allows the body to be centered and the spine to be aligned in positions that avoid stress on the lower back and neck. This is one reason why the system is so safe. Because the exercises are done lying down, the body doesn't have to fight gravity. Not only is the back supported at all times, but any injured area can also be supported while working it. Thus, it is no surprise that dancers, always prone to injury, are fervent advocates of the method, as are osteopaths and physiotherapists.

Although the plié machines are so versatile that you could do an entire class on them – a class involves about 50 exercises – you move on to other apparatus, systematically stretching and strengthening all the muscles in your body. The exercises themselves have a variety of beneficial effects. Firstly, as well as being excellent for overall body toning and firming, they enable you to concentrate on individual problem areas, such as midriff bulge, flabby thighs or stiff hip joints. Secondly, they are designed to give you a beautiful, effortless posture, with tummy and butt pulled in, tension-free shoulders and the merest hollow in your back, rather than a huge sway. Thirdly – and perhaps most importantly – they are extremely effective in reducing tension, stress and anxiety, making you feel happy. This is partly because they make you look good and partly because they are so invigorating to do.

With some of the exercises, you can literally feel the long-term tension floating away. The jackknife exercise is a case in point. This involves doing a kind of shoulder stand, with the aid of a teacher, and then slowly rolling down the backs and legs. This lengthens the spine and massages all the vertebrae as you lower your back, so easing away the tension that has built up in the neck, shoulders and spine.

YOUR OWN PROGRAM

One of the especially valuable features of the Pilates method is the amount of individual attention you receive as you exercise. For the first four or five lessons, the instructor is constantly at your side, making sure that you do the exercises correctly, adjusting the machines to suit your body type and state of fitness, and providing physical support for exercises like the jackknife. This one-to-one tutoring is not only reassuring, it also gives you the necessary confidence and provides an added incentive to persist. I must point out, the body is appallingly lazy, has a short memory and often needs to be prodded into action. Even when you've mastered the equipment and learned the exercises, an instructor should never be far away, correcting you when you go wrong and adjusting the exercises to suit your rate of progress.

Everyone has a different body shape, so I work out a tailor-made program for each of my individual clients. This is designed to allow them to work within their physical capabilities, but also to enable them to achieve their own potential. The key is to always accept what are your actual anatomical limits. No teacher can build on something t hat's simply not there – it's impossible for a short, stocky person to become a long, stringy one, for instance.

People, of course, sometimes have unrealistic ideas about what they want to become, but we're always honest about what we can do. And the exercises we give will get the best possible results out of the shape that God has given them.

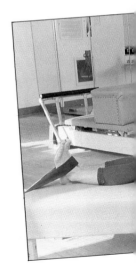

Shape, in fact, is at the core of the Pilates method. Because the system relies heavily on stretching, the end result is the beautiful elongated muscle shape character- istic of the dancer. The dancer's body is basically right. I don't think that a woman cares how much she weighs as long as her body looks good in the mirror. It's inches and proportion that count.

With full body control, inches should be lost from legs, hips, stomach and waist. Thighs and neck should lengthen, the back straighten and the shoulders should

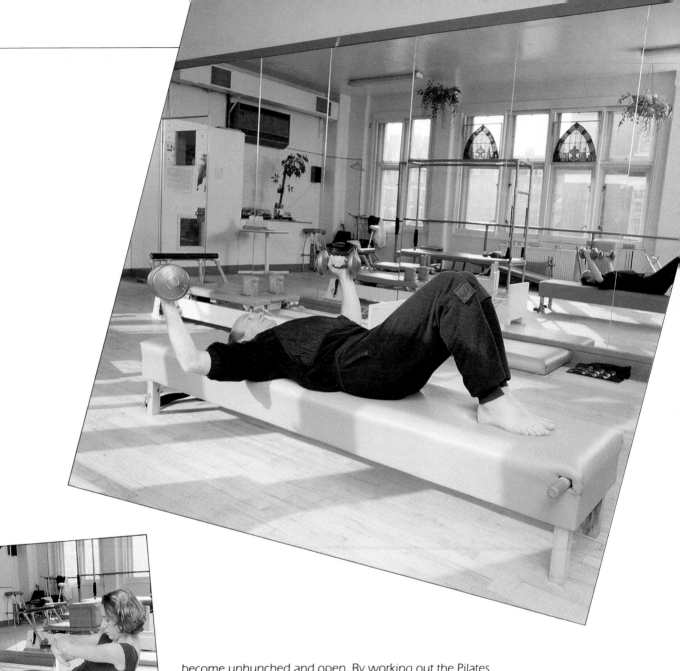

become unhunched and open. By working out the Pilates way regularly, the claim is that you can radically alter the shape of your body, as opposed to many other forms of more violent exercise that may only succeed in building up "bunched" muscles in unwanted areas, so aggravating your figure problem.

Stretching is equally important. Stretching the body is one of the nicest sensations there is. When all the muscles and joints can move freely through the widest possible range of movements, there is a feeling of gracefulness, vitality and freedom, which is one of pure joy. It's difficult to describe, but any dancer could tell you what it means.

BREATHING, MIND AND BODY

In my case, all the body control exercises go hand-in-hand with a special breathing method, borrowed from T'ai Chi. Most people hold their breath when they do anything strenuous, which does nothing except make the task more difficult and encourages the accumulation of tension in their bodies. People come to us after a heavy day and, simply by breathing correctly while they exercise, can dissipate the tension they've been storing.

The idea is that you breathe out as you go into the effort of the exercise and breathe in on the release. Breathing out during the exercise not only helps you to execute it properly; it also elongates the muscles, aids concentration and helps to revitalize the body's energy flow – all essential features of the Pilates method.

Breathing in this conscious fashion helps to promote the state of mental well-being which is one of the core elements of the Pilates method. There is nothing mystical or cultish about it – it is a simple recognition of the German poet Schiller's statement that "it is the mind itself which shapes the body." This, a saying that Pilates himself frequently quoted, is a notion that is being increasingly adopted in both the medical and sporting worlds.

Pilates' idea was that the mind and body should be exercised in union. He was opposed to what he regarded as the automatic limbering of the joints in a conventional work-out program; equally he dismissed the idea of tuning the mind in meditation to the exclusion of the body. By breathing properly as you exercise, you help to bring about this vital integration.

THINKING EXERCISE

Thus, the Pilates method requires concentration. There is no way that you can rush through the exercise program in a fast, sloppy, slap-dash way – you have to think about it. For each and every exercise, there are questions you must ask yourself at all times. Is the back working in conjunction with the thighs, for instance? Is the navel being pushed toward the spine? Is the heel in the right place? Is the neck long? Is the angle of the leg correct? Are you breathing properly?

The Pilates method is the thinking person's exercise technique. You have to work your body as a whole, not just isolated parts of it. When you do this, you begin to become aware of your body as an integrated system. And, when you become really good at it, body control becomes a complete movement study. Far from leaving you mentally drained and exhausted at the end of a class, using your brain in such an intense, focused way serves to promote the wonderful feeling of rejuvenation and stimulation that Pilates' followers rave about. And the mental involvement also eliminates boredom, the scourge of any exercise program.

WHAT YOU NOTICE

It takes around 10 classes for the physical difference to become recognizable. The first change is postural. You begin to stand straighter and start to walk from the hips, rather than the knee, which automatically allows the butt and thighs to start exercising themselves. As the spine starts to return to its proper position and the stomach increases in strength, you naturally "lift" out of your hips. This not only helps you to "walk tall", but shapes up your thighs. When you begin to stand correctly, the tension on the neck and shoulder vanishes and tension in the lower back also disappears. An intergral part of any good exercise program is the cooling down, or relaxing, period. Indeed cooling down is just as important as warming up your body before you start the main part of any routine.

When you relax, what you are aiming to do is to help your body adjust to a less strenuous level of physical activity. This is why what is termed "pacing" in exercise is vitally important – you should never push yourself beyond your physical limits. What you need is to have some energy in reserve for the equally important relaxation exercises. These exercises are deliberately gentle. They are designed to help your heart rate to return to normal and to protect you against any bodily stiffness.

So, anyone can work out the Pilates way – my pupils, for example, range from 12-year-old schoolgirls to 75-year-old grandmothers. Actors work out to improve their body awareness and to gain the strength to help them to cope with long, arduous parts. Physiotherapists and osteopaths send patients who need help to ease joint problems. And ordinary men and women – housewives, secretaries, businessmen – come simply to stop feeling sluggish, shape up and to start feeling their muscles again. All you need is the requisite patience, sense of involvement and the belief that shaping up and working out is good for you, in both physical and mental terms.

The Nautilus alternative

The Pilates system, with its emphasis on gentle, gradual exercise, is closely linked to the home exercise programs outlined in the main sections of this book. However, there is nothing to stop you combining the toning programs given here with contrasting class exercises, provided that you understand clearly what the latter have to offer. Take the increasingly popular Nautilus system, for instance. Nothing could be further removed from the quiet and calm of the typical Pilates workout – or of the home workout programs described later in this book – than the bustle of a Nautilus studio. Yet you can combine both forms of exercise to benefit your body.

What immediately catches the eye in a Nautilus studio are the gleaming, sophisticated, highly fashionable black and chrome exercise machines, designed to exercise just about every muscle in your body. These have changed the face of weight training for thousands of women.

Nautilus started in the mid-1970s, when the American designer and weight trainer Arthur Jones decided to devise a program to improve body building. Along with countless other athletes, he knew that, in any exercise movement, certain parts are easier to perform than others. This meant that, by definition, the muscles could not be worked uniformly – at one stage, for instance, a muscle would be working at its maximum, while at others it would be grossly underworked. What was needed, he decided, was a piece of equipment that would work the muscle equally hard throughout all its range, thus making training programs more effective.

NAUTILUS IN ACTION

Jones therefore came up with his now famous excercise machinery, which is based around the operation of a special cam. This is a type of pulley, which, when linked to a system of weights and levers, varies the resistance the machine offers to the exerciser. These means, in theory, that a muscle can be worked throughout its full range.

What does this mean in practice? You sit, lie or stand in the appropriate machine in the correct position and exercise a specific part of your body, using the appropriate weight for your state of fitness.

To select the weight you require, you simply adjust a steel pin in the weight stack attached to the machine. As you get fitter, you move the pin a notch at a time down the weight stack, thereby increasing the load against which your muscles are working. The weights run along

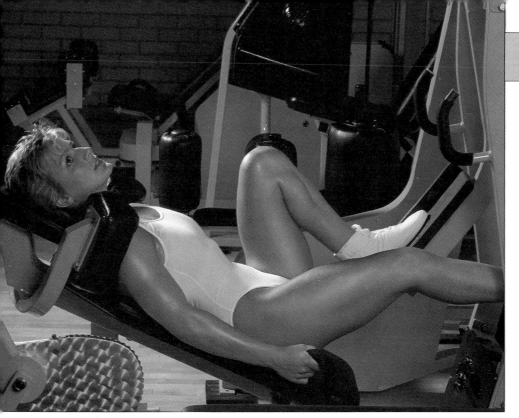

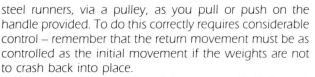

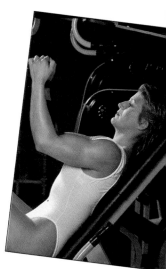

steel runners, via a pulley, as you pull or push on the handle provided. To do this correctly requires considerable control – remember that the return movement must be as controlled as the initial movement if the weights are not to crash back into place.

What does this type of weight training offer? Firstly, it is very good for toning the body and reaching muscles that other systems cannot easily exercise – one machine, for instance, is designed to exercise the inner thigh. Secondly, it is a safe method, in so far as the weights cannot drop on your head, or your toe. However, you can injure yourself if you sit or lie in the wrong position while you work out (even though a belt is provided to hold you in the right place, this does very little to correct bad postural habits). So, proper supervision is vital, which is why it is important to find a bona fide Nautilus gym or sports club in the first place.

In a well-equipped gym, there should be Adductor and Abductor machines for inside and outside thighs, machines to exercise the back of the arms, a machine for the waist, a machine for the butt muscles and backs of the thighs, a machine for stretching the hamstrings and a machine to firm up the pectorals, the muscles that hold up the bust, among many others. Some machines, however, are designed solely for male use; the "shrug machine", designed to build up the trapezius muscle into the no-neck look favored by body builders, is a typical example.

WORKING OUT THE NAUTILUS WAY

To get any tangible result from Nautilus-type equipment, you need to exercise three times a week for at least a 10- to 12-week period, each training session lasting about an hour. It takes four to five sessions to learn how to use all the machines properly and to feel at home with them; after this, it takes another two to three weeks for the body to learn what the equipment is teaching it to do. By the third or fourth week, you should be realizing that you can really achieve something and your self-esteem and self-image will start to improve. Over the following weeks, this should increase still further, as your muscles become more defined and your general fitness accelerates.

Though you may not actually lose weight, you'll probably lose inches, as your body fat starts to fall away. If you're worried about becoming muscle bound, make sure that your training program is structured accordingly. This is especially important if you are stocky; stocky people tend to put on muscle bulk more easily than other body types.

NAUTILUS WATCHPOINTS

Before you start working out the Nautilus way, check out the following points:

● Make sure that you are taken around the gym at least three times by a qualified instructor and get him to explain and demonstrate the equipment to you. You must ensure that you know how to use it.

● Make sure that the gym takes your health profile before embarking on any training. This should include checks on any past injuries, muscle and joint problems, general medical history, blood pressure, body flexibility and lung capacity.

● Your training program should be tailored to meet your needs. Make sure that it is balanced. There should be a variety of programs from which to choose – figure improvement, increased stamina, muscle definition, weight increase, strength improvement, and overall fitness. Ideally, you should be given a chart, so that you can monitor your progress. This acts as an incentive and as a helpful motivating force when the going gets tough.

● Every conscientious gym supervisor should know enough about your physiology and anatomy to be able to tell you with total honesty what you can and cannot achieve.

● Remember that no Nautilus equipment on its own can turn you into a superman or superwoman. You have to put in the work.

At the start, each exercise needs at least 12 to 15 repetitions (these should increase, along with the weights, as you progress). If you cut down on the repetitions while increasing the weights, you will only encourage muscle bulk. And, before you even start on the machines, you must allow for a 10- to 15-minute warm-up period. It is essential to do this before you try the machines, as your muscles and joints will be looser and so less prone to strain and injury.

Try jogging on the spot, working out on a cycle machine (all well-equipped gyms should have one of these), or ask the instructor to devise you a series of suitable exercises. Whichever method you choose, all movements should be rhythmic and controlled.

When you start using the equipment, remember that it is essential to breathe correctly while working with the weights. You should breathe out as you lift and in on the release (your instructor should ensure that you do this).

If at any time you feel sick, dizzy or in pain, stop immediately and get off the machine. Learn to listen to your body – it always knows what is best for you.

Your training program should be changed regularly to keep in line with your progress and to eliminate the risk of boredom. The latter is one of the biggest negative factors in weight training, although, in a Nautilus gym, this is often offset by pop music and the sight of other people working out.

Most important of all, make sure that the gym you choose is a responsible one and not just in the business to make a fast buck. An instructor should be on the floor watching you all the time and you should be encouraged to develop a rapport with him or her, so that you feel free to ask questions or seek advice whenever you feel it necessary. Such advice and instruction should be given willingly and as promptly as possible. With this type of intensive physical training, you need personal attention right through the program, not just at its beginning. This is vital as it will ensure that the most effective and safest program of Nautilus training as possible is given to everyone who wants it.

Note: It is important when exercising weights that you proceed carefully to avoid injuring yourself. If you have not been exercising regularly, start the exercises without wearing weights. If you have problems with your back or any joints, be especially cautious. And exercise particular care during any exercise in which the arms or legs are extended away from the body. At the first sign of strain during any exercise, STOP. Consult your physician before continuing with the program.

Your 30-minute Routine

The 30-minute work out that follows this introduction forms the core of your personal body toning program. It is intended to help to stretch your muscles and to shift those excess pounds. By following through the exercises in sequence, you will soon find how stimulating the program can be; as you progress, you will find that your mind is being toned as well and you will sharpen up mentally as well as physically as a result.

Before you start, remember these basic points. Never, ever, over-stress your body, especially if you are unaccustomed to exercise. This is why you should work through the routine without the weights at first; only add them when you feel ready to do so. Similarly, do not try to beat the clock; the 30 minutes is only a guideline – it is not a rigid target.

If you find a specific exercise or exercises a strain, stop. To help you, each exercise is graded according to level of difficulty, a single star indicating the least demanding level and so on. Finally, never let the program become boring – if it becomes a chore, it will have failed in its purpose.

This 30-minute routine is designed to work systematically through the muscles of every part of your body, so it forms the daily basis for your fitness program. You can practice the routine at any time, but it is particularly good for waking your body up in the morning. Though this may come as a surprise to you, it is a fact – as many experienced exercisers will tell you – that a good exercise routine actually leaves you feeling that you have more energy, not less!

In addition to the exercises in this basic program, you can incorporate any of the other exercises in this book into the routine, provided that your body feels ready for it. Indeed, you should include new exercises as soon as you can, since all routines benefit from variety.

If you have not been exercising regularly, start by working through the routine without weights and cutting down on the number of repetitions given for each exercise. Then build up gradually to the full routine, using weights on the easier exercises – these are marked with a single star – and then progressing to the tougher ones (those marked with two or three stars), until you are using weights throughout the whole routine.

Do not worry about how long this takes you. What is important is that you progress in gradual stages, taking on only as much extra weight as you are ready for, so that your body is not put under excess strain. If you ignore this golden rule, the results could be dangerous.

The other important point to remember is that you should try to make your routine as fun and exciting as possible.

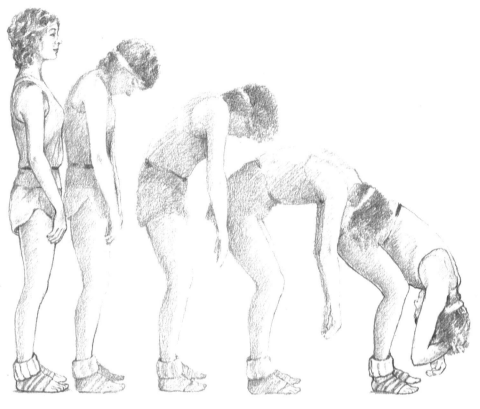

EXERCISE 1 ✳

The first stage of the routine stretches your body gently, giving your muscles time to warm up. The first exercise warms up the all-important spinal column.

1 First, think about your posture. Stand up straight with your feet about 18 in. (45 cm.) apart and slightly turned out, your shoulders dropped and relaxed, your head in line with your spine. Your body should feel lifted; there should be space between the ribs and the pelvis, which helps counteract any overarching in the small of the back. Wearing the weights on the ankles reinforces posture

and helps you to feel a continual lengthening of legs and spine.

2 Now drop the head down on to the chest for eight stretches. The neck is curved, but not shortened.

3 Take the curve further into the shoulders and chest. The waist does not bend at this point, but the knees should have some "give" in them – don't hold them tensely. Eight stretches.

4 Take the curve into the waist and drop down with more bend in the knees for a further eight stretches.

5 Now let the whole body take up the bounce and drop down from the hips, coming as close as you can to your bent knees, but without forcing – remember that this is only a warm-up and you should not be straining. Eight stretches.

6 Roll the body slowly upwards into the correct postural position. As you come up, feel the buttock muscles working to anchor the base of the spine – don't let your stomach or your butt stick out! Try to feel the legs lengthening out of the hip sockets and each of the vertebrae placing itself above the one below. Make sure that the stomach is held in

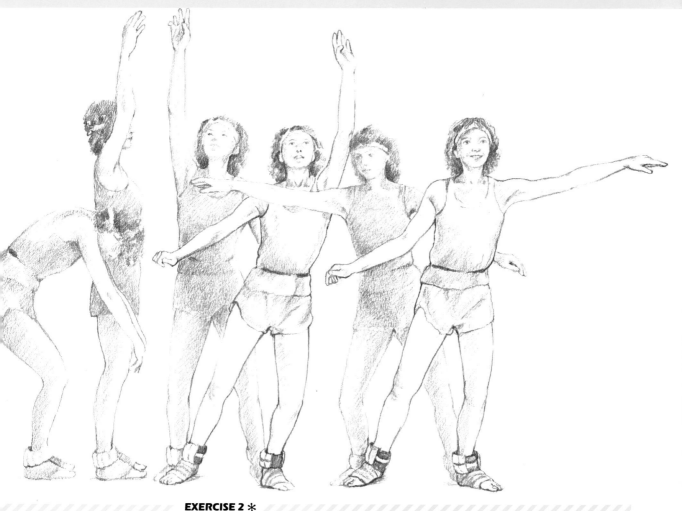

EXERCISE 2 ✳

and back towards the spine. The head comes up last.

7 Now take your extended arms up in front of your body, so that they make a V-shape held slightly forward of your shoulders. Stretch up through the body and into the fingers. There should be air between the ribs and all of the body should feel lifted. This does not mean, though, that your shoulders are hunched up – the arms should be lifted from the middle of the back, not by displacing the shoulder. The neck is long and the gaze is straight ahead – don't look up to the ceiling.

Do the whole exercise twice.

1 Stretch alternate arms up to the ceiling. Bend the knee on the same side as the lifted arm you are stretching, shifting your body weight from side to side.

2 Make sure that your arm goes straight up – it should never bend back from the shoulder. The arm should move from the shoulder blade; the shoulder itself should be pulled down into the back. This is not just an arm stretch – the top half of the body should be reaching up out of the waist. Repeat 16 times.

3 Stretch in the same way as you did before, but this time take your arms out to the side instead of upwards.

4 Again, make sure that the arm is held from the back and your shoulder is dropped. Your ribs should lift up and out to the side. You should feel them reach all the way up the side and out along the arm as one long stretch. Repeat 16 times.

31

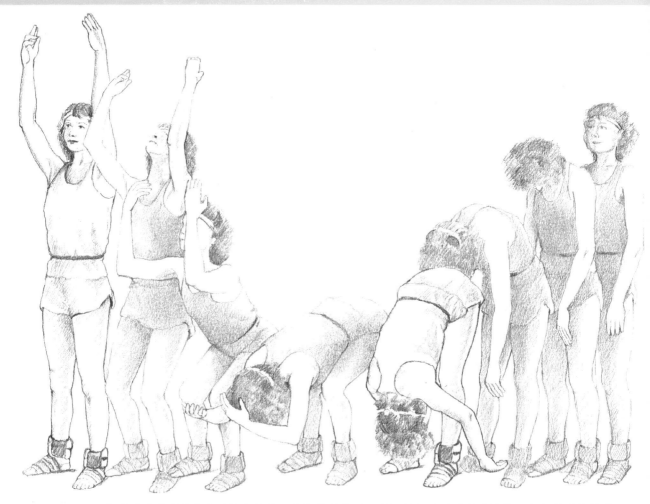

EXERCISE 3 ✳✳

Here, in a movement borrowed from contemporary dance, you take the stretch right through the body and ripple back up at the end to perfect posture.

1 Take up the same standing posture as at the start of the routine. Then lift both arms up and above the head, palms facing you, and look up towards the ceiling, feeling your whole body and legs stretched.

2 Now bend your knees and elbows and begin to curl downward, allowing your back to curve slightly. Keep your gaze up for as long as you can.

3 As you curl down, let your gaze drop to the floor. Keep your arms straight in front of you, palms upward.

4 Keep curling down until your chest touches your thighs.

5 As soon as your chest has made contact with your thighs, start to straighten your legs, keeping your chest touching your legs for as long as possible. Then straighten your legs completely, so that your body is hanging down from the waist. Check that there is no tension in your neck and shoulders – you should be hanging loosely, like a rag doll.

6 Now start to uncurl slowly back to a standing position. Uncurl vertebra by vertebra, feeling each one fall into place on top of the last, as in the first exercise. Start with a pelvic tilt.

7 Let your arms and head hang loosely until your neck and shoulders have uncurled.

8 You should now be standing straight with a slight pelvic tilt, leg muscles pulled up, buttocks and stomach lightly held in, shoulders down and looking straight ahead. Do the whole exercise four times.

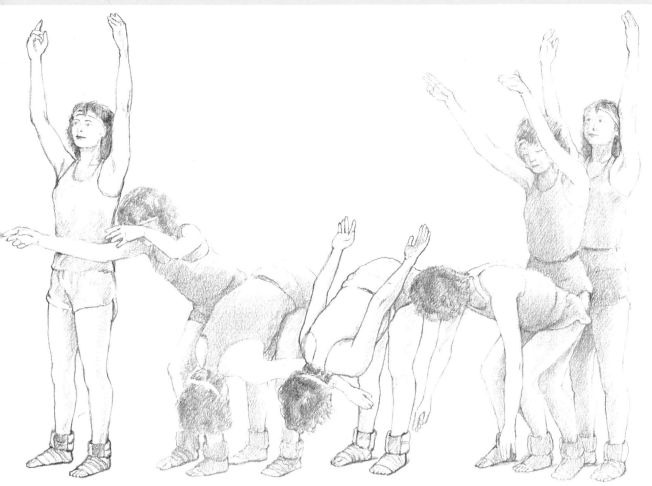

EXERCISE 4 *

This last warm-up speeds up the ripple down of Exercises 1 and 3 – though this doesn't mean you can skimp any part of it.

1, 2 With the arms held up, palms facing, bend the body at the hips and, in one long sweep, take the chest down towards your knees, which start to bend as soon as the movement begins.

3, 4 As your chest reaches your knees, straighten the legs and take the arms back behind you, your upper body hanging down from the hips. The whole movement should be smooth and quick, with your arms describing a wide arc.

5, 6, 7 To return to a standing position, you repeat the exercise in reverse. Check your posture when you get back to the standing position – your knees and legs should be pulled up, your stomach and buttock muscles held in, the ribs held up with lots of air in between them and the shoulders dropped down into the back. Eight times right through.

33

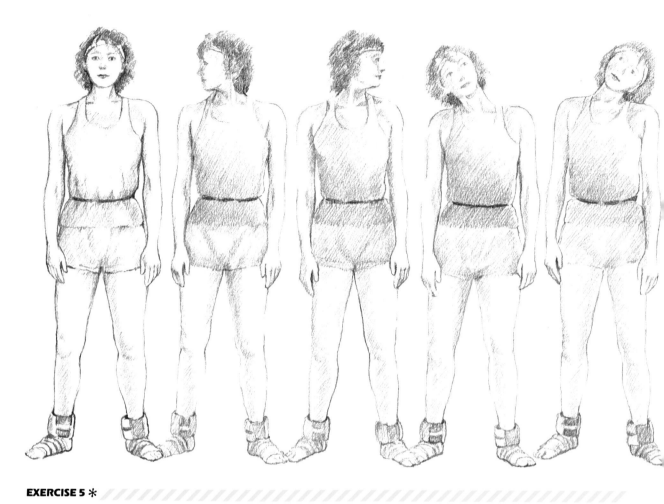

EXERCISE 5 ✳ ///

The neck and shoulders are the seat of much of the body's tension; the following exercises are designed to release this and get them both moving. It is important to ensure that only the head and neck physically move – not the shoulders.

1 Take up the correct posture, standing up straight with your feet about 18 in. (45 cm.) apart.

2 First, turn your head to look over your right shoulder, aiming to line up your nose with the shoulder. If you feel your shoulder starting to tense, reduce the amount you turn.

3 Repeat, this time looking to the left. Eight times each side, alternating.

4, 5 The head now drops down to the side – you should feel a good stretch up the long side of the neck. As in the first part of the exercise, it is the neck that is working – make sure that the head is going down to the shoulder, rather than the shoulder being lifted up to the ear! Eight times each side, alternating.

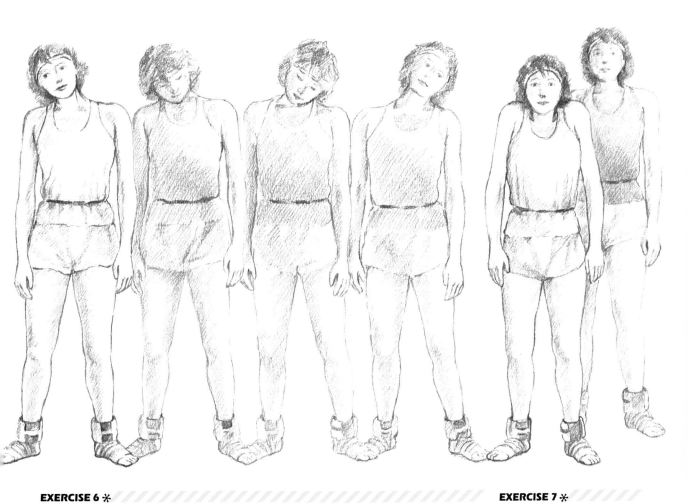

EXERCISE 6 ✳

1, 2 Drop the head down to the right and let it roll round in a semi-circle to the left, **3, 4**.

Repeat, starting on the left. Four times each way.

EXERCISE 7 ✳

1, 2 At last, the shoulders are allowed to move up towards the ears! Lift them right up and then let them drop down heavily. Feel how your neck lengthens when they are in the down position. Eight times.

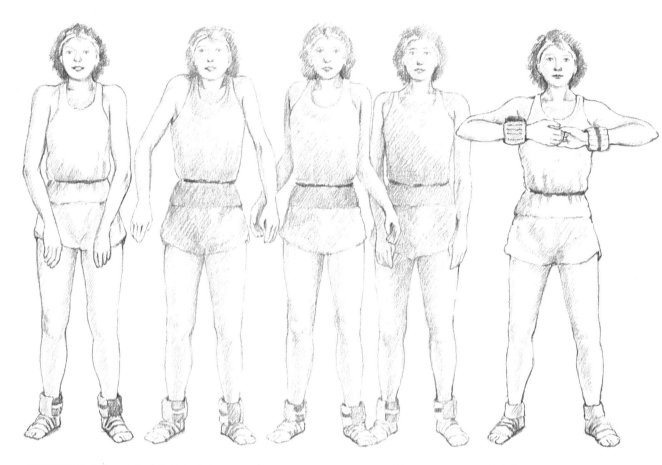

EXERCISE 8 ✶✶ ///

1 The shoulders now make a square. Starting in the dropped position, take them forward first. If you are doing this correctly, the arms will have turned in the sockets, so that your palms are facing away from you.

2 Now lift the shoulders up to the ears, as in the last exercise.

3, 4 Then pull the shoulders down and back, so that your shoulder blades squeeze together. Finally, drop them right down. If you feel any tension in the neck drop the head forwards; and remember to correct any overarching in the small of the back, especially when you take the shoulders back. Four times right through, making the movement a fluid one if you like – a circle rather than a square.

EXERCISE 9 ✶ ///////////

1 Transfer the weights to the wrists. Standing in the same postural position as for the last exercises with the feet 18 in. (45 cm.) apart, clasp the fingers together in line with the chest. Now pull the fingers away from each other without actually letting go. You should feel the muscles of the upper arms working together with the pectorals as the chest opens. Eight times.

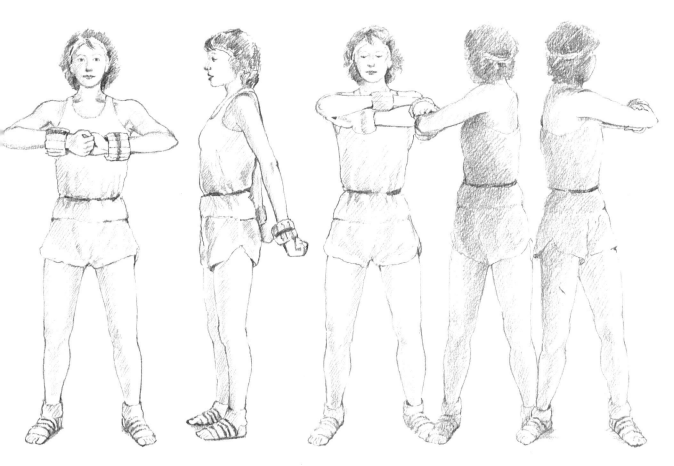

EXERCISE 10 ✳ //////

1 This is the same exercise in reverse – this time the hands push together. In both this and the previous exercise, the head should be lifted, with the neck long. If your neck feels tense, drop the head forwards to the chest. Eight times.

EXERCISE 11 ✳✳ /////

1 This is quite a strong exercise for the back and upper arms. Take the arms straight back behind you, with the backs of the hands facing towards each other. When you get the arms back as far as you think they will go, try to push them back just that little bit further. Check that you're not overarching in the back – it takes a lot of work with the stomach and buttock muscles to stop this. Again, if your neck feels tense, drop the head on to the chest. Eight times.

EXERCISE 12 ✳ /////////////////

Throughout this exercise, it is important to ensure that the turn comes from the waist. The hips should face the front at all times; neither they nor the knees should move.

1 Standing with your feet 18 in. (45 cm.) apart and your knees slightly bent and facing front, fold your arms in front of you so that your right hand rests on your left elbow and vice versa.

2 Now, turning from the waist, turn right to look over your shoulder with eight little pushes round towards the back.

3 Pass through the center and repeat with eight on the left side. Repeat again, with four on each side and then two.

37

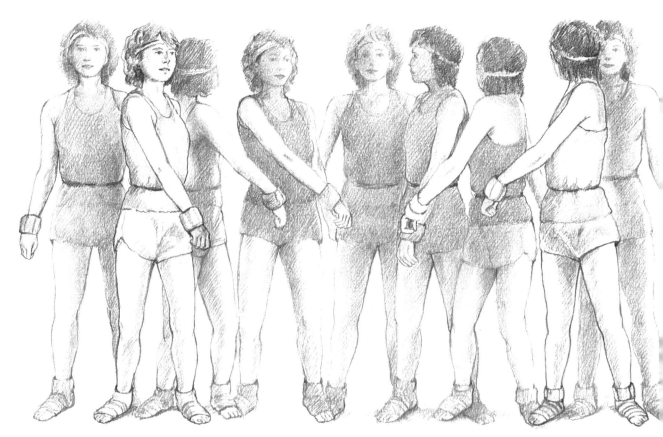

EXERCISE 13 ✳ ///

This exercise is a continuation of the previous one, the difference being that the arms now swing round freely.

1, 2, 3 Stand with straight legs and start to turn from the waist to the left, letting your knees bend as you do so.

4, 5 As you come through the center, your knees straighten again.

6, 7, 8, 9 You bend again as you continue to circle round to the right. This is an easy sweeping swing where only the upper body moves – the knees and hips face front all the time. Eight times, alternating.

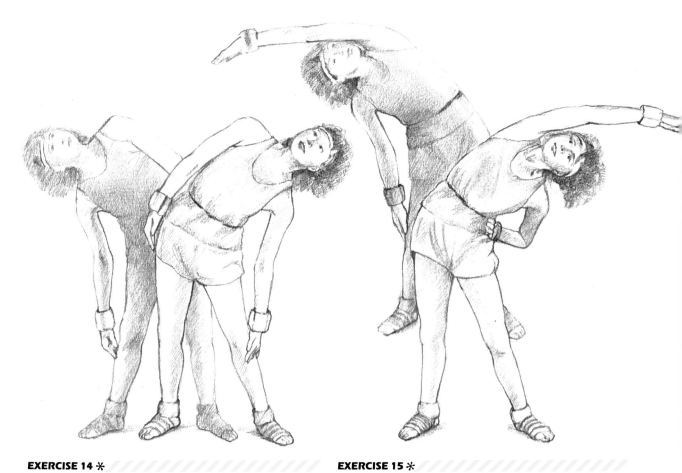

EXERCISE 14 ✳ ///////////////////////////

The next two exercises take the waist stretch down the side.

Stand in a good postural position with the feet little more than a hip width apart.**1, 2.** Drop down your right side, the hand sliding down the leg. Let your upper body curve over, feeling the head as a heavy weight, and stretch all the way up the left side. Keep your hips still and centered – don't let the left one jut out to the side. Eight each side.

EXERCISE 15 ✳ ///////////////////////////

1, 2 Dropping down your right side as in the last exercise, take your left arm over your head and stretch it out to the side, the upper arm in contact with your face. This is a harder stretch – the weight on your upper arm will take you further. Again, take care not to move your knees or hips. Eight each side.

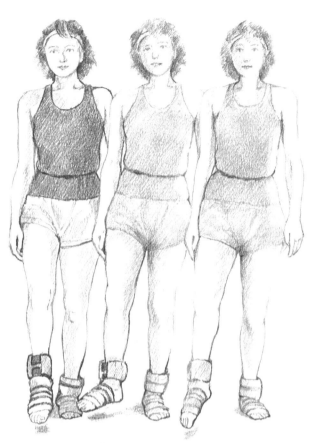

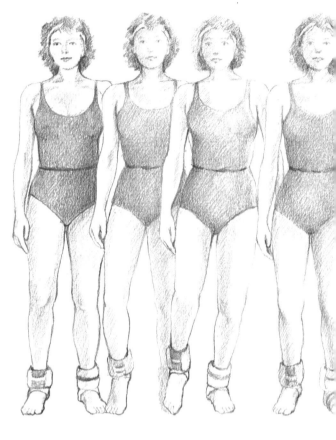

EXERCISE 16 ✳✳ //////////////////////////

Transfer the weights to the ankles. The legs and upper body should now be warmed up, so, before you start the short running/stamina section of the routine, you must do the same for the feet.

If you find balancing difficult initially, you can rest your hand on the back of a chair. However, it should not be difficult to keep your balance if you hold your center of gravity by pulling up your stomach muscles and buttocks.

1 Standing with your feet together, take the right one forward, pointing your toes.

2, 3 Now circle the foot from the ankle, circling clockwise and then counterclockwise eight times. Repeat on the left.

It is worth practising your balance by holding a rise on your toes. If you are holding your muscles correctly, you should be able to stay there practically for ever!

EXERCISE 17 ✳ //////////////////////////

1, 2, 3 Go through your feet, transfering your weight as you lift up your right heel, the instep, the ball of the foot and finally the toes.

4, 5, Put your weight down again in the same way. Then repeat the entire exercise on the left. Eight times, alternating.

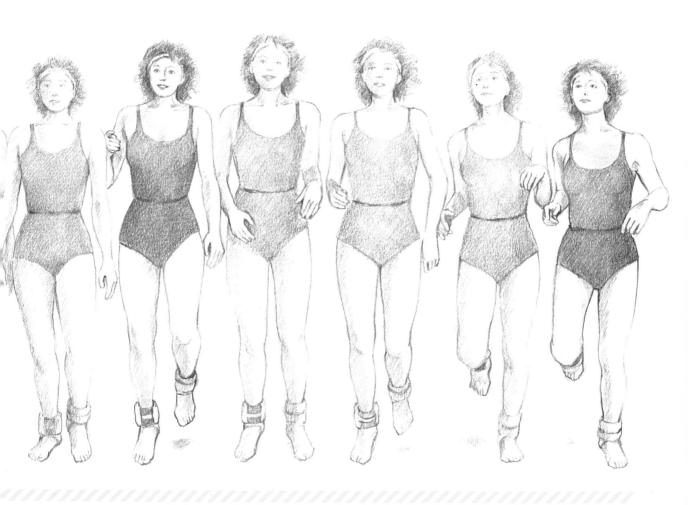

6-10 Now speed up so that you break into a gentle run, arms relaxed, for about one minute. Don't try the entire turning sequence at first – build up gradually, but always end with the gentle running and ripple through the feet. If you stop suddenly, you may get cramps. Make sure that your knees are always directly above your feet, as there is a tendency for them to turn in as you tire.

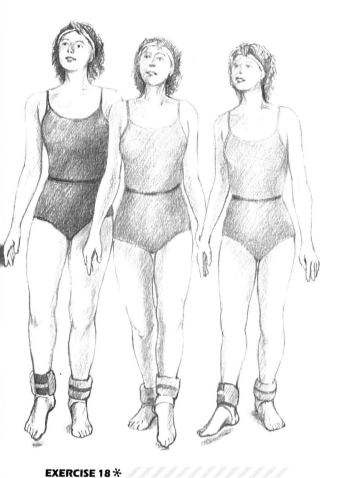

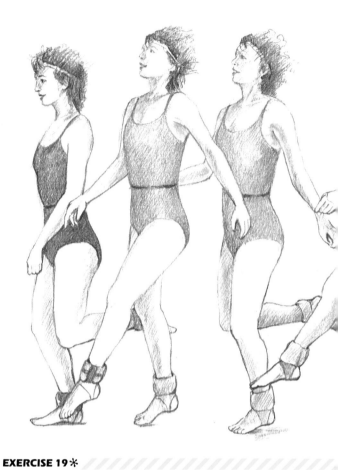

EXERCISE 18 ✳

1, 2, 3 Keeping to the same
rhythm as before, point the feet
forward instead of taking them
back into the run. 32 times,
alternating.

EXERCISE 19 ✳

1, 2, 3, 4 Using the same
gentle kicks as in the last
exercise, add a hop between
them. Do one hop and one kick
on each side, alternating 32
times, letting the arms swing
gently with the movement.

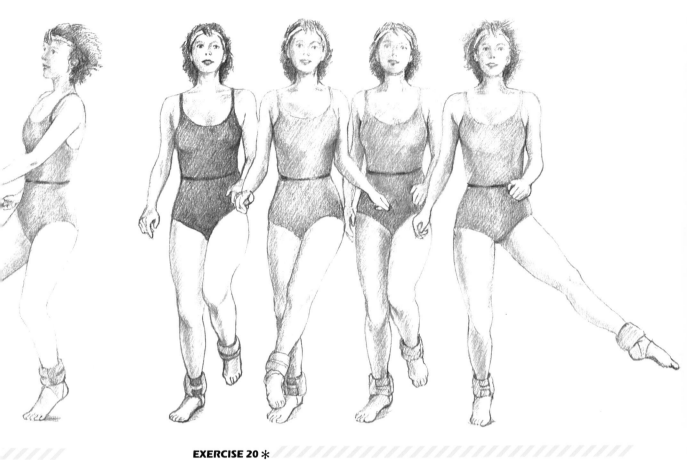

EXERCISE 20 ✳

1, 2, 3, 4 This time, add a sideways kick to the exercise, so that the pattern is hop, kick forwards, hop, kick out to the side. 32, alternating.

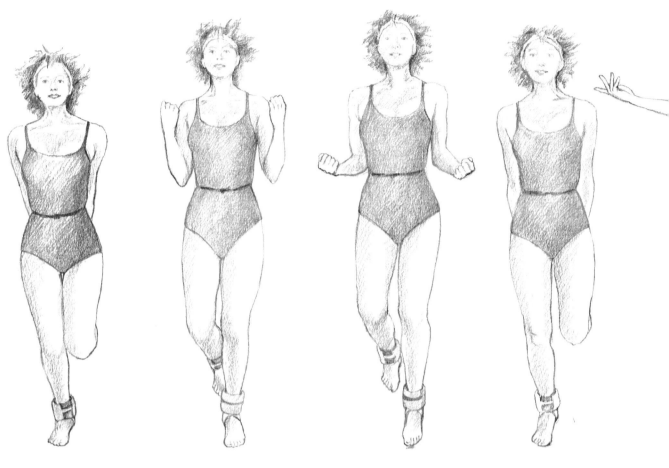

EXERCISE 21 ✳ ///

1 Revert to gentle running, making sure each time that you go right through the feet, so that the heels touch the floor and that the knees are directly above the feet, not rolling inwards.

2, 3, 4 Folding your arms at the elbows, bring the fists up to the chest and then down past your sides, taking the arms straight out to the back as far as they will go. The arms should rotate with the movement, so that the backs of the hands pass the thighs and the palms face the chest when the arms are raised in front of you. 32 times.

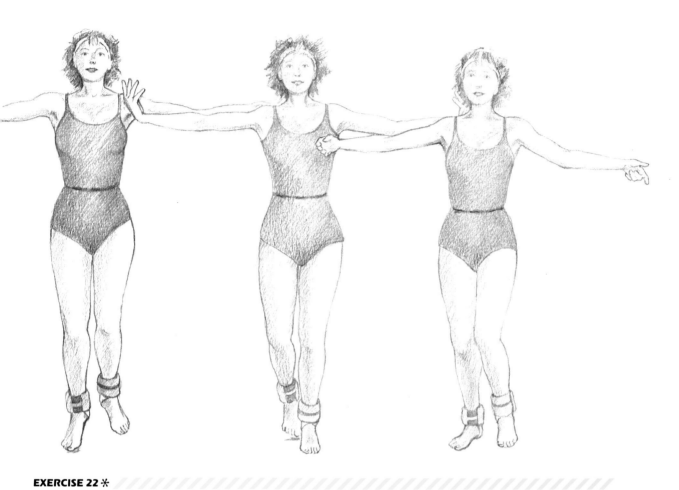

EXERCISE 22 ✳ //

1, 2, 3 Running gently – *again,
don't forget the feet* – take the
arms straight out to the side at
shoulder height. Keeping the
shoulders still, rotate the hands
from the wrists 16 times
clockwise, 16 counterclockwise.
If your neck or shoulders are very
tense, drop your head forward.

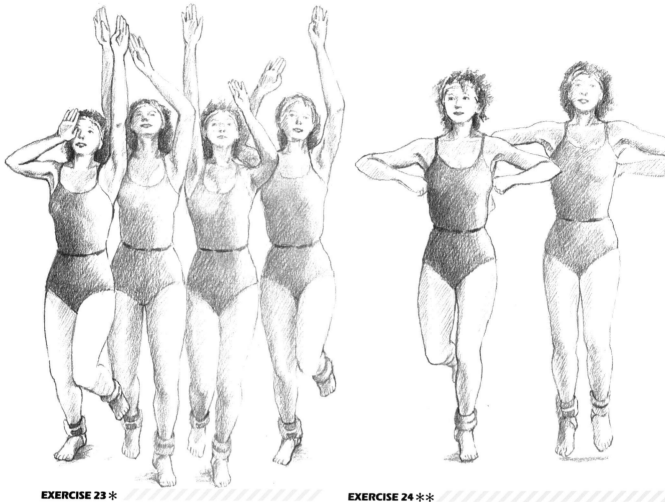

EXERCISE 23 ✳ ///////////////////////

1, 2, 3, 4 Still running, stretch up the arms alternately above the head. You should feel your whole body stretching right through to the fingertips. Look up to the ceiling to your outstretched hand. 32 times, alternating.

EXERCISE 24 ✳✳ ///////////////////////

1, 2 Carry on running if you can, though you can walk through this exercise if you prefer. Make sure that you are still using the feet fully, and that the knees are directly over the feet, not turning inward. Stretch out your arms to the side in line with your shoulders.

3, 4 Bending the arms at the elbows – the upper arms and shoulders don't move – let your fingertips describe a full semi-circle as they come into your chest. In and out 32 times.

46

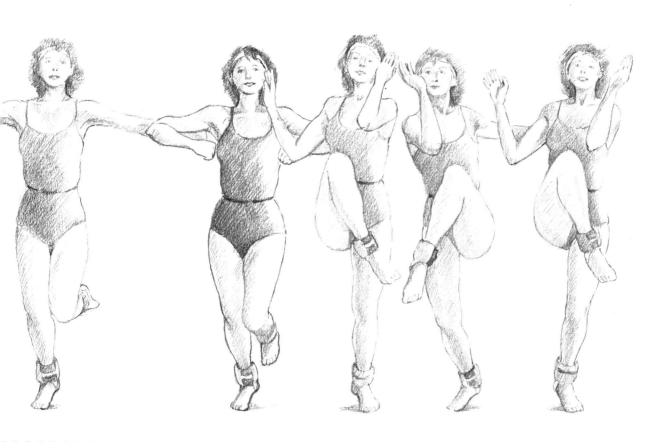

EXERCISE 25 ✳✳

1, 2, 3 Hopping from leg to leg takes your knee up towards your chest and brings the opposite elbow down to meet it. It is vital that it is the leg that is coming up – not the upper body coming down – so keep your back straight! 32 times, alternating.

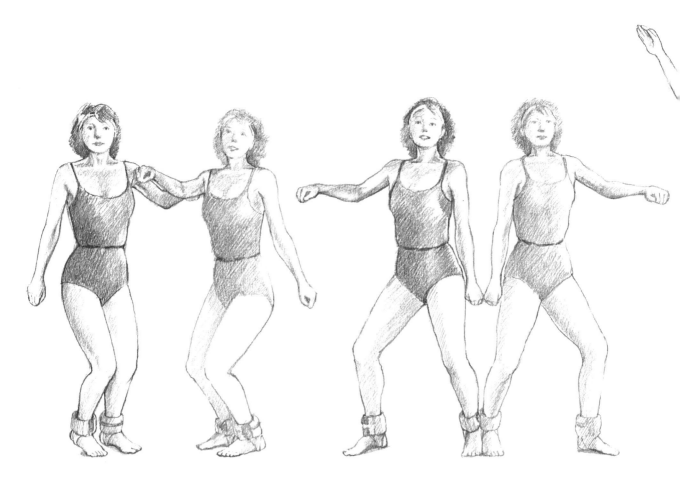

EXERCISE 26 ✳ ///////////////

1, 2 These little jumps with the
feet together twist the upper
part of the body in the opposite
direction to the lower part, so
that your feet turn away from
your head and you feel a good
stretch right through the body,
especially at the waist. Let the
arms follow through in a swing
in the same way as the
shoulders. 32 times.

EXERCISE 27 ✳ ///////////////

1, 2 Do the last exercise again,
but this time with the feet apart
instead of together. Feel the
thrust of the twist coming from
the buttocks.

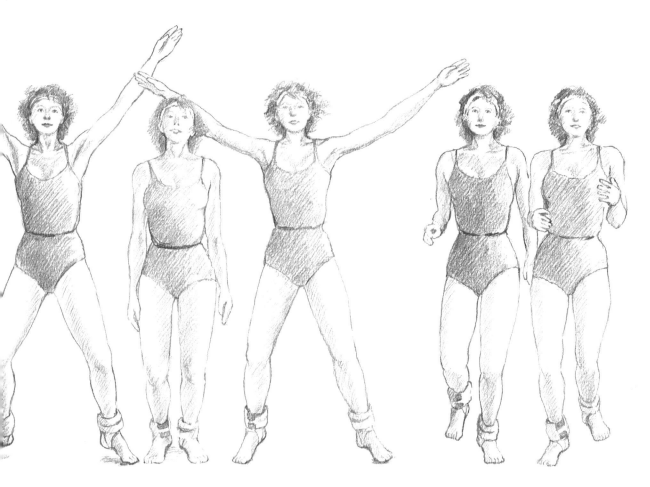

EXERCISE 28 ✳ ///////////////////////////////////////

1 These are star jumps. From a central position of the feet together and slightly turned out, jump the feet out, raising the arms at the same time to make a star shape.

2, 3 Whenever the feet are on the ground, whether together or apart, the heels should be down and there should be a little "give" in the knees. As in the last exercise, the buttocks should be doing a lot of the work. 32 times.

EXERCISE 29 ✳ //////////

1, 2 Now start slowing down, running gently, making sure that the feet go down properly each time. Slow down gradually to a walk.

49

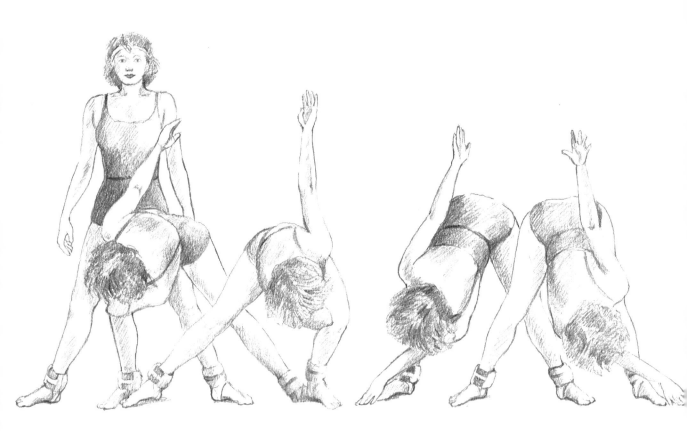

EXERCISE 30 ✶ /////////////////////

1, 2, 3 Now that the body is completely warmed up, you can really stretch it out. Standing with the feet slightly turned out and 3 ft. (1 m.) apart, the tailbone tucked well in, bend the right knee, dropping the left elbow down to it. The upper body turns toward the right knee and the right arm is lifted out behind to extend the stretch still further. Staying low, bend the left knee and take the right elbow down to it. 16 times, alternating.

EXERCISE 31 ✶ /////////////////////

1 This exercise follows on from the last without rising up in the center. So, staying low, keep the legs straight and stretch the opposite hand down the front of the leg.

2 Eventually, your aim is to get the hand on the floor the other side of the foot, but don't strain for this. Let your body go at its own pace – it will get there in the end. 16 times, alternating.

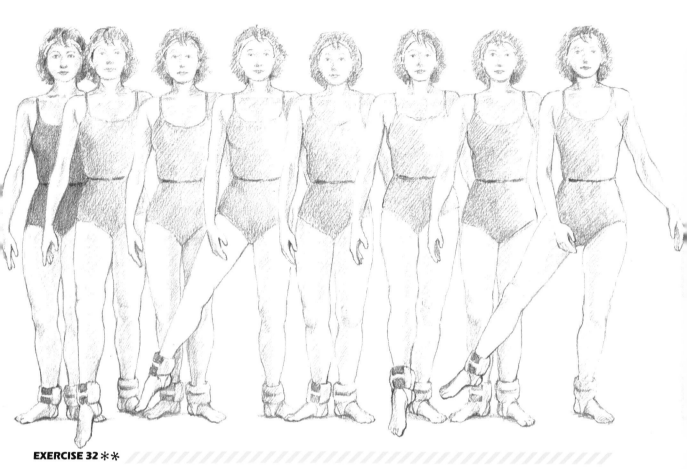

EXERCISE 32 ✳✳

1 Hold the body in a good posture, with pulled up legs, tucked in butt, stomach muscles lifted, the shoulders dropped into the back with the arms held a little way out from the sides to give the chest an open feeling, and the head balanced on top of a long neck. The legs and feet are turned out – but the turn-out comes from the top of the legs in the hip socket. Never turn out your toes further than your knees can go. When you bend (or plié), the knee should always be directly above the foot.

2 These next exercises may appear easy, but, in fact, they are very hard work, if you are doing them properly. With a pointed toe, take the right foot straight out in front of you, really reaching out of the hip socket. Keep your balance by holding your center in your stomach and buttock muscles – these are never allowed relax until you have completed the exercise.

3 The main part of this movement is not the pointing out but the drawing back in, so pull the foot in slowly, feeling the movement in both the buttocks and the thigh muscles. Pull the foot back to a central

standing position, checking that you have not allowed your hips to be thrown out of line – no re-adjustment should be necessary! Four times on each leg.

4 Now, take the foot straight out to the side in the turned-out position – your knee should be facing the ceiling. Again , the major part of the movement is the pulling in. This time, it is the muscles of the inner thigh that do the work.

5 As you come back to center, check that the stomach and buttock muscles are pulled up and you are not tensing up in the neck. Four on each leg.

6, 7 Repeat the whole exercise, with the foot coming slightly off the floor. This means that you must concentrate even more on your pulled-up stomach, as otherwise you will lose your balance or compensate by leaning into a hip. As you take the leg out, really extend it as far as it will go, stretching out the whole leg and foot. Four times on each leg.

8 When you go to the side, don't try to lift the leg too high. Make sure, though, that the knee is facing the ceiling and, as in all the stages of this exercise, the buttock muscles are pulled in hard. Four times on each leg.

51

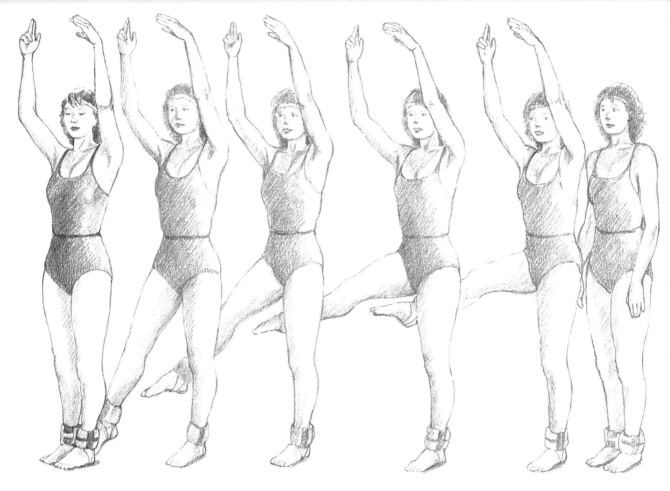

EXERCISE 33 ✳✳✳ /// **EXERCISE 34** ✳✳

1 This is a very tough exercise to do properly. Stand in a well-held posture, the arms lifted so that the hands are slightly forward of the face, and check that the spine is completely in alignment – this means a slight pelvic tilt. The feet are parallel. Don't forget that, though the arms are lifted up, the shoulders are down and held strongly in the back.

2 Now extend the right leg straight in front of you, lifting it slightly off the ground and feeling the whole leg stretch. Then draw it back to the central parallel position. This is a slow movement, so you need to hold in the stomach and buttock

muscles to retain your balance. Make sure that this concentration doesn't tense your shoulders – there should be lots of air in the upper body.

3 In the next movement, the leg is lifted a little higher. Check that the knee is still parallel to the ceiling throughout.

4 The leg now comes up higher still; however, do not sacrifice the straightness of your spine or your balance for height.

5 The last movement takes the leg to its highest point. Again, check that it is the leg alone that moves – don't shift your weight to make the movement easier. Work through the whole sequence twice (alternating) on each leg.

The next series of exercises is the plié, taken in three of its various positions. This is one of the most important exercises in both classical ballet and contemporary dance. It may look like a simple knee-bend, but it is, in fact, a complex movement, when performed properly. The weights act mainly as reminders for placement, as the feet remain firmly on the floor. In none of these pliés should even the heels come off the floor.

1 The first plié is in parallel position, the feet together and pointing directly ahead. It is vital that your posture is correct right from the start, so check that your

52

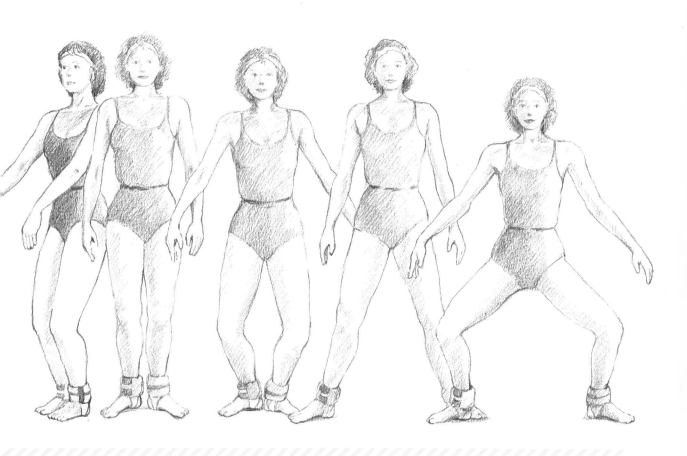

legs are straight, and that your knees and the muscles of your thighs are pulled up. Feel your spine as long as possible and absolutely straight. To achieve this, hold your stomach in with the buttock muscles tucking under to help posture. The upper body is held straight and tall, with the head held high and not tilted.

2 As you breathe out, bend your knees as much as you can without taking your heels off the floor, at the same time ensuring that your back stays absolutely straight. You should feel your stomach muscles pushing back toward your spine and the spine

itself growing longer. Imagine that you are growing taller with the movement, so that, even though your knees are bending, it is as if you are aimimg to keep your head on the same level! Breathe in to come up again, concentrating on keeping the spine completely in line. This will mean pulling up your buttock muscles hard. Four slow pliés.

3 The next plié is in first position, the feet making a V-shape. Don't try to turn out your feet too much. Your knees should be directly over your feet when you bend. If they're rolling in, change the position of your feet. Your

legs and spine are pulled up, as in the parallel plié, but, in this open position, your thigh muscles "wrap round". You should feel as if your inner thigh is trying to face front! This also means that the buttock muscles are pulled right under, too. The combination of these muscles and the stomach working together gives a real feeling of strength – even if someone pushed you, you shouldn't waver if you are doing the exercise properly.

4 The movement here is exactly the same as for the parallel plié. You bend the knees as you breathe out, at the same time

lengthening the spine. They come up as you breathe in.

5 The last of the pliés is in second position, the feet about 18 in. (45 cm.) apart.

6 Again, make sure that the knees are directly over the feet when you bend them. The muscles work in the same way as in the last exercise, the thigh muscles wrapping round, the inner ones pulling toward each other as you come up. It can be even harder to keep the back straight in this position – check sideways in a mirror to make sure that you're not arching. Four slow pliés.

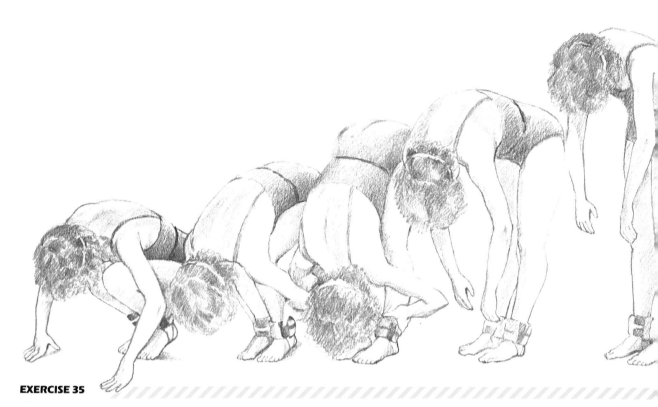

EXERCISE 35

1 These stretches are similar to those at the beginning of the routine, though now your body is warmed up, you can stretch it out more. Start with your body flat against your thighs, heels off the floor, hands on the ground in front of you. Do four little stretches in this position, keeping your body glued to your legs.

2 Now put your heels on the floor, but keep your chest glued to your thighs, holding on to the backs of your ankles. Four stretches.

3 Ideally, you should keep the legs in this position with the upper body flat against them. However, if you can't manage this, just keep your body against your legs and straighten them as much as possible. Four stretches.

4, 5, 6 Now roll up through the back, vertebra by vertebra, until you are standing in an erect, held posture. Don't forget that the head comes up last – it isn't lifted until the final stage of the roll-up. Check that you haven't tensed your shoulders.

Repeat the whole sequence four times.

54

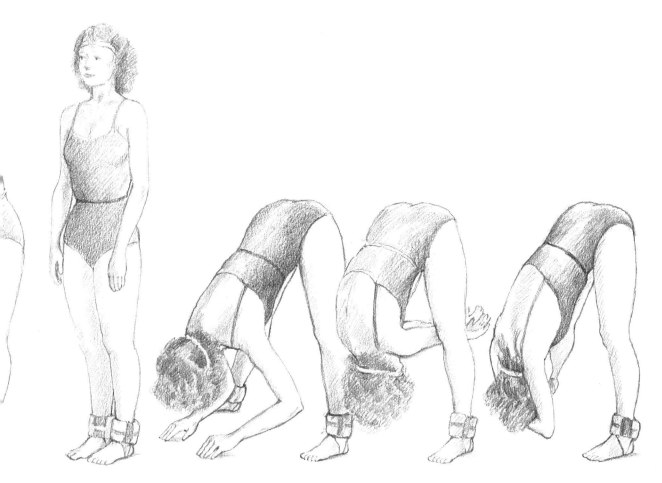

EXERCISE 36 ✱

1 Stand with the feet about 1 m. (3 ft.) apart, with your legs straight. Drop down, hands on or towards the floor, feeling the stretch through the legs. In this exercise the head is acting as the weight. Eight stretches.

EXERCISE 37 ✱

1 Stay in the same position, but now reach through your legs for further eight stretches. Alternate between the two positions, 16 stretches in all.

EXERCISE 38 ✱

1 In this exercise, simply hang down in the same position as in Exercise 36, folding your arms to add to the weight of your head. Hold the position for about 30 seconds, feeling your spine iron itself out as it relaxes.

55

EXERCISE 39 ✳

1 Sitting on the floor, stretch one leg out in front of you, knee to the ceiling, foot pointed. Bend the other at the knee, with the foot of this leg against the opposing knee. The extended leg should be stretching as far forward as possible. Sit up as tall as you can.

2 Hinging at the hips and keeping the back absolutely straight, reach forwards down the extended leg toward your pointed foot. Your head should be in line with your spine, while your arms, though stretched, should be reaching from the center of the back – avoid any hunching of the shoulders.

3 Here, you are ideally aiming to lay the upper body down the leg, but this will take time. At the start, just remember to keep the back straight, resisting the temptation to round the back in an attempt to get lower. Eight reaches on each leg.

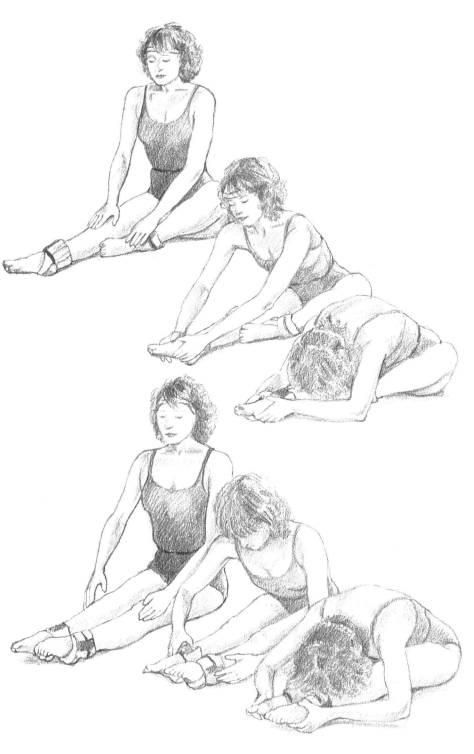

EXERCISE 40 ✳✳

1 This exercise is slightly harder than the last one, since both legs are straight out in front of you. Again point the feet and really extend the legs as much as you can. If you clench your butt muscles, you will find yourself sitting up about two inches taller – try it.

2 Reach forward as before, hinging at the hips with a flat back, shoulders down and into the back.

3 Again, you are aiming to lie flat against the leg, but don't sacrifice your straight back to get lower – this will come in time. Eight reaches.

56

EXERCISE 41 ✳✳

1 The last of these exercises is the hardest one. This time, the knees are again facing toward the ceiling, but the feet are flexed. If your leg muscles are really working, your feet should be off the floor, the backs of your knees pressing down hard. Again, don't forget your sitting muscles!

2 Reach forward down the leg with a flat back. Your stomach should be lifted, but don't transfer any strain to your neck or shoulders.

3 In this position, you will find that you will not be able to get down as low as in the others. The vital point is to keep the back flat. You can grab hold of your legs or ankles to pull you down a bit further, but don't pull hard enough to strain yourself. Eight reaches.

EXERCISE 42 ✳✳✳

1 Lying flat on the floor with knees stretched out and facing the ceiling, feel the whole length of your back long and flat against the floor. You will have to press your navel toward your spine to feel this.

2 Now lift the leg up, so that your toes reach out and up toward the ceiling. Though the leg is stretching out, most of the work in this exercise is done by the stomach muscles, which have to press hard into the floor to prevent the back from arching. Try not to tense the shoulders and keep the lower leg stretched out as well.

3 Keeping the leg stretched out, take it as far as you can in an arc toward the face. Then lower it to the floor, again pressing the navel into the spine. Four lifts on each leg.

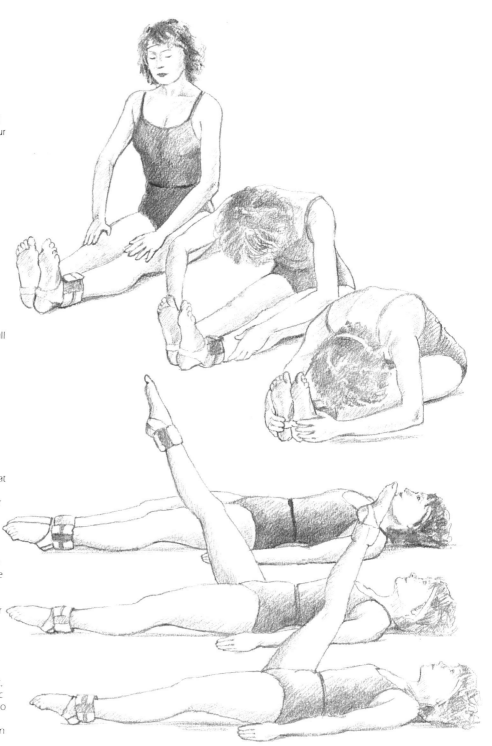

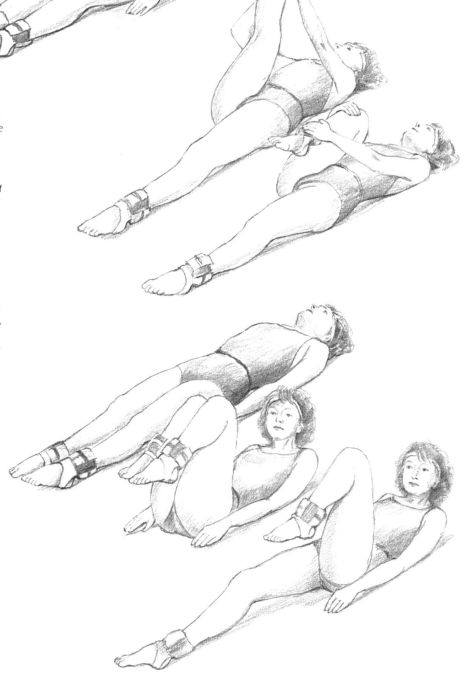

EXERCISE 43 ✳✳

1 In the same position as for the last exercise, stomach pushing back toward the spine, feel your body lengthened out against the floor.

2 Raise one leg, extending it as far as it will go, foot pointed. Again, don't let the back arch off the floor. Take hold of the leg or ankle with both hands and gently pull the leg towards you. Check that the other leg is also stretching out and its whole length is pressed to the floor. Four stretches.

3 Now bend the leg at the knee and then, with one hand on the knee and the other on the ankle, pull the leg to the body. Four times. Lower the leg to the floor.
   Repeat the whole sequence on the other side.

EXERCISE 44 ✳✳✳

1, 2 Starting in the same flat position as in the last exercise, draw the knees up to the chest and then curve the head and shoulders up from the floor. The arms are stretched out low against the sides. The chin should be dropped right down on the chest.

3 Now stretch out one leg, keeping it close to the floor. Really feel the leg pulling away from the body, extending right out from the foot. Draw the leg back in and extend the other one. Alternate, eight on each side, keeping the body curved up throughout.

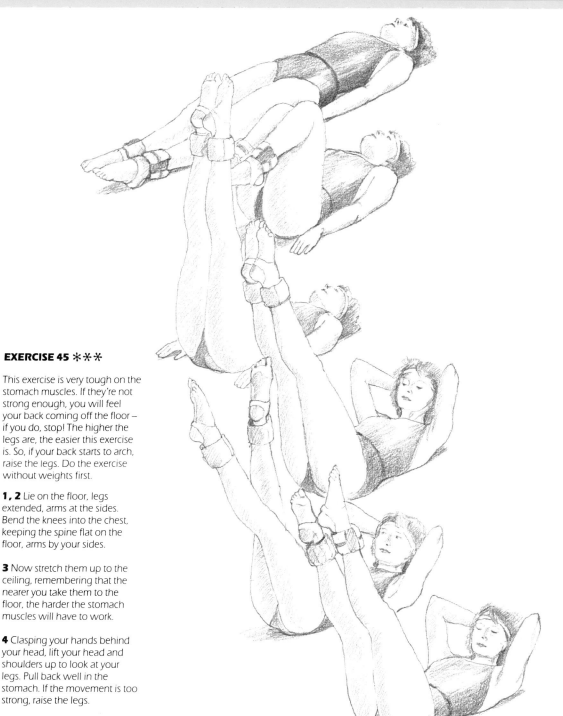

EXERCISE 45 ✳✳✳

This exercise is very tough on the stomach muscles. If they're not strong enough, you will feel your back coming off the floor – if you do, stop! The higher the legs are, the easier this exercise is. So, if your back starts to arch, raise the legs. Do the exercise without weights first.

1, 2 Lie on the floor, legs extended, arms at the sides. Bend the knees into the chest, keeping the spine flat on the floor, arms by your sides.

3 Now stretch them up to the ceiling, remembering that the nearer you take them to the floor, the harder the stomach muscles will have to work.

4 Clasping your hands behind your head, lift your head and shoulders up to look at your legs. Pull back well in the stomach. If the movement is too strong, raise the legs.

5, 6 Now scissor your legs, crossing them at the ankles. Try not to tense in the shoulders or neck. 16 scissors.

EXERCISE 46 ✳✳

1 Lie on your side, propped up one elbow, the other hand in front of you on the floor for balance. The lower leg is bent and the foot is flexed extended top leg with a flexed foot up toward the ceiling, the heel pushing hard away from you the whole time, pulling the leg out of the hip socket. To keep a straight back, you will need to keep a firm hold of your stomach muscles. Check that the back is in alignment by doing this exercise against a wall. The leg is raised quite high to start with, so that the lifts themselves are quite small, but you should feel them right through the leg and even into the waist. 16 on each side. Then making the movement bigger, point the foot and lower it to be in line with your body. Flexing hard, lift as high as you can. Eight each leg.

EXERCISE 47 ✳✳✳

1, 2 This is another exercise which works the stomach as well as stretching out the leg, Start by taking up the same position as for the last exercise, but this time take your upper leg forward, so that it is at a right angle to your body. Flex hard and hold on to your stomach! Eight lifts each leg.

EXERCISE 48 ✳✳

1 This exercise is a combination of the previous two. Lie on your side and raise the extended top leg, flexing hard and pushing away from the hip as before.

2 As you take the leg down, bend the knee and bring it into your chest.

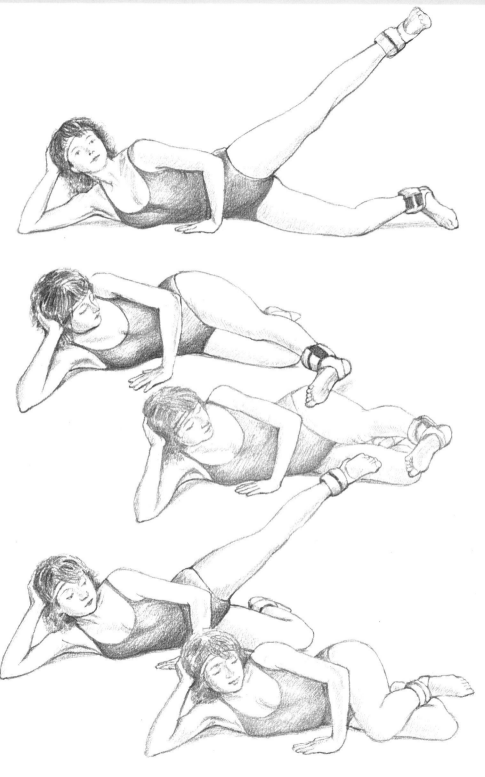

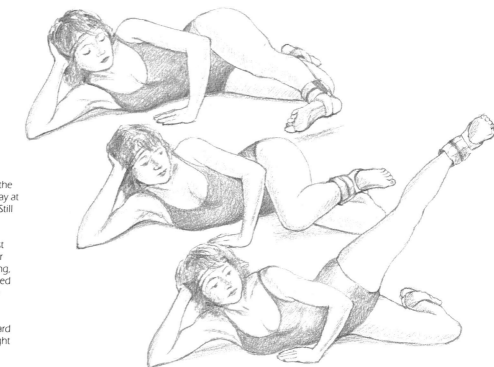

3 Now unfold the leg from the knee, so that it stretches away at right angles from the body. Still flex hard.

4 Bend the leg into the chest again, making sure that your stomach muscles are working, so that your back is not arched or wobbling about with the effort of the movement.

5 Now take the leg up toward the ceiling again. Repeat eight times on each side.

EXERCISE 49 ✷✷

1 This exercise is for the inner thigh muscles. Lie along the floor, the body raised on an elbow. Cross the upper leg in front of the lower thigh, holding on to the ankle with the top hand. Keep the upper body straight during this exercise – don't let it sink into the ground.

2 Flexing hard and pushing the heel away, lift the lower leg off the floor. This is not a big movement – you will not be able to lift the leg more than a few inches from the floor. Eight each side. Now try the movement again, pointing the foot.

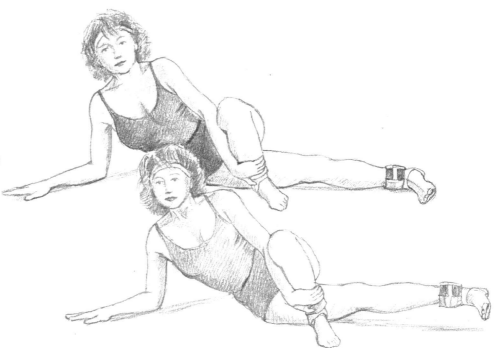

61

EXERCISE 50 ✳

1 Lie on your front, your face on your hands, which you should cross in front of you. Bend the underneath leg slightly and keep the foot flexed. Raise the other leg, pointing the foot and extending the leg as far out as it will go. You should be able to feel the leg muscles working right into the butt. 16 lifts each side.

EXERCISE 51 ✳

1 At the furthest stretch of the last exercise, flex your foot.

2 Now bend the leg back with the foot still flexed, keeping the knee itself completely still.

3 Extend the leg out again, still with a flexed foot, and see if you can raise it a little higher each time you straighten it. Four each side.

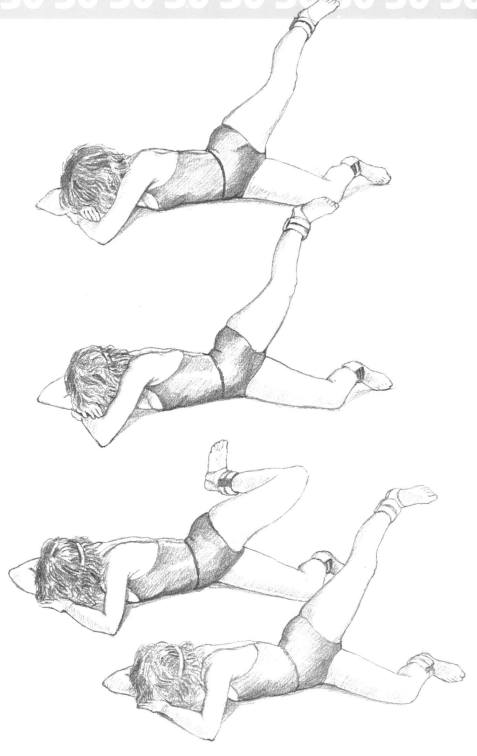

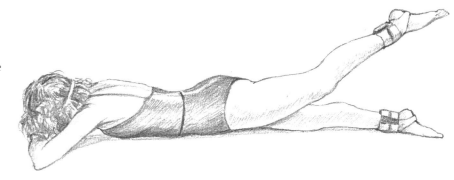

EXERCISE 52 ✳

1 Lie flat on your front, your face on your arms, as before. Raise one leg behind you as high as you can and, in that position, make 16 little circles with a pointed foot, circling clockwise and then counterclockwise. Repeat on the other leg.

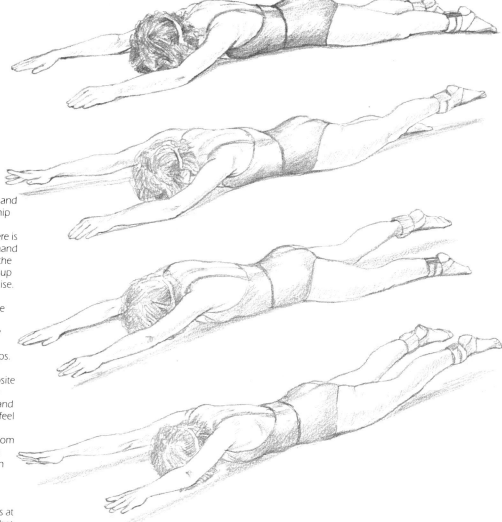

EXERCISE 53 ✳✳✳

1 Lie flat on the floor, facing down. Stretch out your arms and legs, with your feet about a hip width apart. Pull up your stomach muscles, so that there is enough space to slide your hand between your stomach and the floor. Try to keep that pulled-up feeling throughout this exercise.

2 Stretch out one arm and the opposite leg simultaneously. Feel the stretch right the way through the body out to the pointed toes and the fingertips.

3 Now repeat with the opposite arm and leg, still keeping the stomach muscles pulled up and the shoulders relaxed. Try to feel as if there were actually someone trying to pull you from each end to make the stretch fully extended. Eight times on each side.

4 Now repeat the exercise, stretching both arms and legs at the same time. Don't forget that the stomach is lifted! Eight times.

EXERCISE 54 ✳✳✳

1 Arch up from the floor, stretched legs raised with pointed feet and arms stretching out in front of you. Your head and chest are off the floor as well. Now tap your feet together, working up to 50 taps.

EXERCISE 55 ✳

1 This position gives you the chance to recover after all your hard work! Kneel down, body along the thighs, head on the floor, arms alongside the legs, palms uppermost. Breathe deeply, relaxing into the pose for about 30 seconds.

EXERCISE 56 ✳✳

These next exercises are all based on a contemporary dance movement, the contraction. This may look simple but, like the pliés, it involves your entire body.
1 With the weights on your wrists, lie on the floor with a slight pelvic tilt, your legs stretched in front of you, arms by your side.
2 Pull the stomach muscles back toward your spine and the floor, tightening your buttock muscles under you at the same time. This will cause your knees to bend slightly and your chest to come up a little from the floor. This is not visibly a big movement, but, as it uses the center of your body, it is essential that you get it right before you start rolling up from the floor. Four times.

EXERCISE 57 ✳✳

1, 2 Make sure that you are working your body in a good contraction, as shown in the last exercise, before you start this one. Moving with the contraction, lift your upper body off the floor, arms outstretched and parallel to the floor. Your head comes last, dropping behind you like a heavy weight. Do not come far enough to

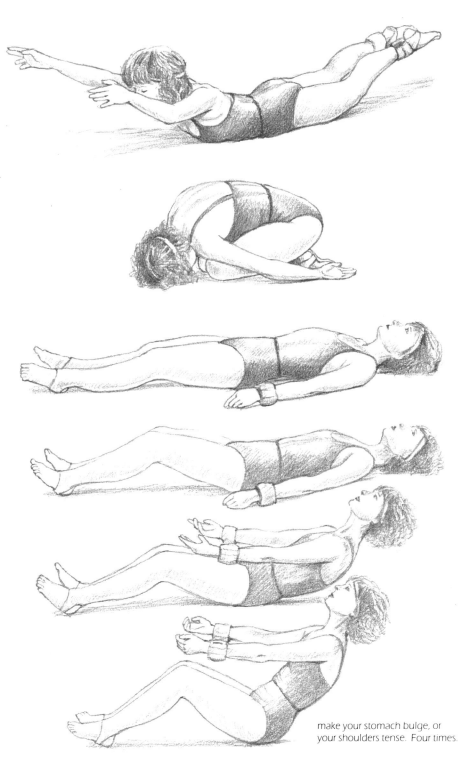

make your stomach bulge, or your shoulders tense. Four times.

EXERCISE 58 ✳✳✳

1 The third stage of this exercise should be attempted only when you are certain that your stomach muscles are strong enough to carry it out correctly. As before, go into your contraction on the floor before you start the upward lift.

2 Curve up, maintaining the contraction and stretching out your arms. Make sure that there is no tension in the neck or shoulders and that the head is heavy.

3 Roll up in the contraction until you are sitting straight up, arms stretched out in front of you. When you get to the top, lift your head, placing it in a straight line on top of your spine. Release.

4 Now drop the head forward, so that the chin is on the chest, and start to roll down through the spine, taking up the contraction again. As you change direction and start to move down toward the floor, soften the chest and let the rounded quality of the movement go into the arms, so that they curve. Your palms should face downward.

5 Holding the contraction, gently roll the back down. You should feel each vertebra touching the floor in turn and lengthening out the back.

6 Lying down, feel the spine really stretched out along the floor, the legs extending with pointed feet. Four times through.

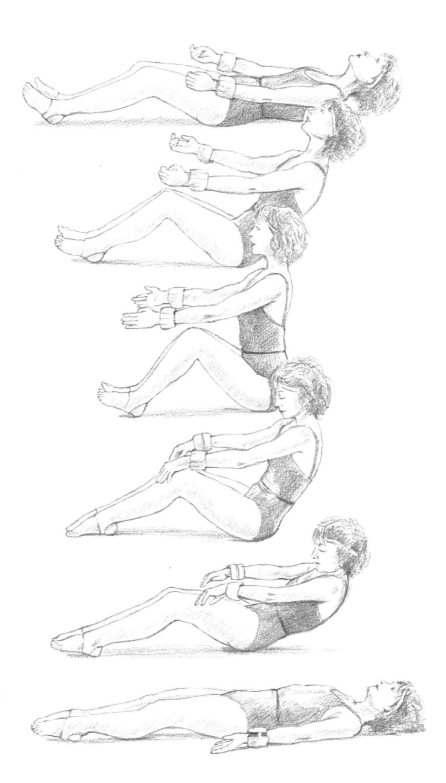

EXERCISE 59 ✳✳✳

1 This exercise is also based on contracting the stomach muscles, but is even harder, as it depends on holding one position. Start by lying flat on the floor and contract the stomach muscles so that you start to come up from your starting position.

2 Roll up until you are about half-way to a sitting position, knees bent, arms outstretched in front of you. Loosely clench your fists, then raise one arm above your head, which is lifted in this exercise, not dropped back.

3, 4 Take the lifted arm straight down in front of you as you raise the other one. This is just like pulling a rope. The movement is very hard on the stomach muscles, so make sure that they can take the strain. If they bulge out or quiver, sit up higher. Eight pulls.

EXERCISE 60 ✳✳✳

1 This is a further stomach-contracting exercise – and another very tough one. Roll up into the same position as the one you used at the start of the last exercise. Make loose fists.

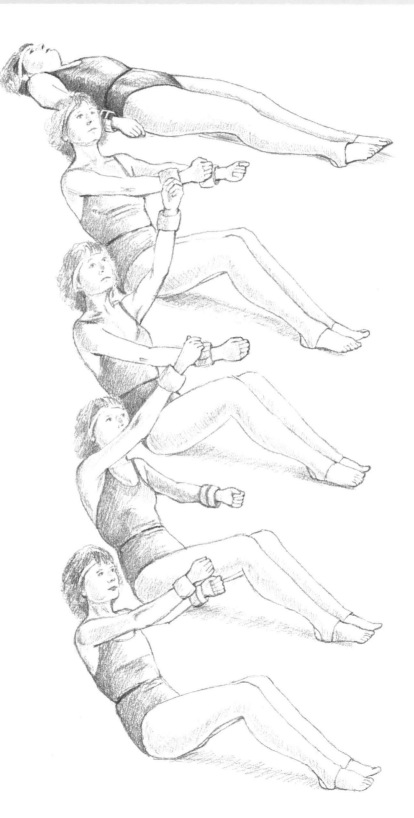

2 Crossing one fist above the other, raise your arms until they are reaching up toward the ceiling, taking care not to tense the neck or the shoulders. If it seems that they are taking the strain, drop your chin down to your chest. If this fails to relieve the strain, leave this exercise until your stomach muscles are stronger.

3 Now reverse the movement and, in four crosses, bring the arms down again. Repeat the whole sequence, four times up and down.

EXERCISE 61 ✳

1 Transfer the weights to your ankles and sit up with your legs fully extended in front of you, feet pointed. Your back should be straight, your arms stretched out straight from the shoulders and you should be sitting up tall on tight butt muscles.

2 Maintaining exactly the same position, flex the feet hard, the knees still pointing up at the ceiling. If you're pushing away sufficiently, your heels will come off the floor. Point and flex eight times.

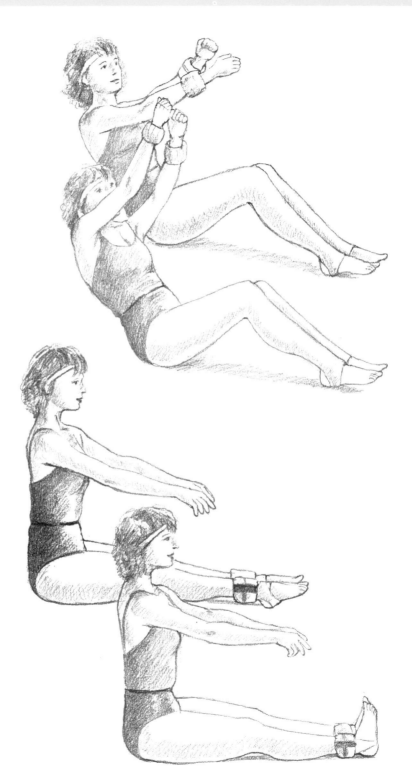

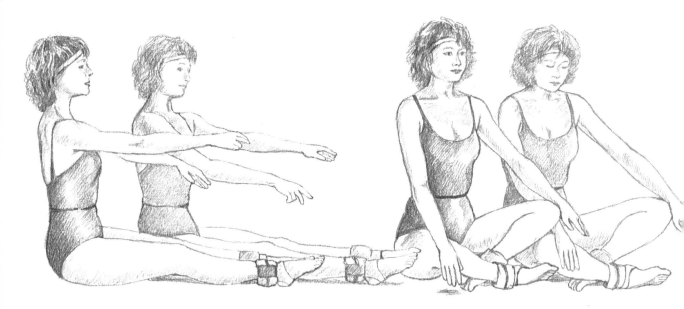

EXERCISE 62 *

1 Take up the same starting position as in the last exercise. Stretch out your arms straight in front of you, sitting tall, feet pointed.

2 Moving the right leg first out from the hip, make eight little "walks" forwards. Repeat, but this time moving back. Do the whole movement twice.

EXERCISE 63 *

1 Sit cross-legged, your hands resting on your knees. Before starting the main stages of the exercise, check that the neck and shoulders are free from tension by rolling your head in a gentle semi-circle from side to side. Now sit up tall, arms stretched out beyond the knees.

2 Using the same contraction as in the earlier exercises, pull the navel against the spine, tightening the butt and wrapping the thigh muscles round, so that the legs should drop down a little lower. The back will curve and the head should follow its line, so that you will be gazing down toward the floor. The chest and shoulders are very soft and open in this movement, and both should be free from tension. Eight contractions, sitting up to release between each one.

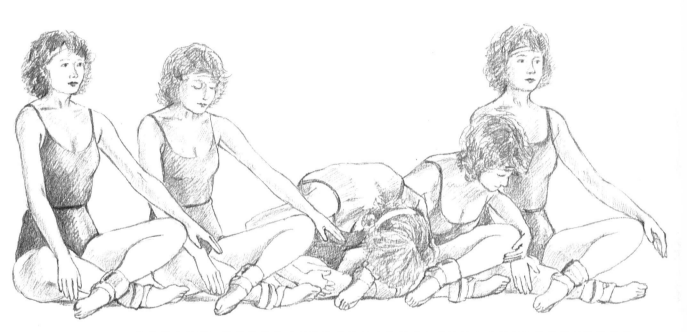

EXERCISE 64 ✳✳

1 This exercise is a development of the last one. Re-cross your legs, so that the other foot is in front, and sit up very tall.

2 Contract as before, pulling the abdominal muscles back to curve the spine.

3 Take the contraction forward in one piece, so that the head reaches forward and down to the ankles. The hands clasp to the knees.

4 Straighten out the spine, releasing the contraction until your back is absolutely flat, your head in line with it. The base of your spine should not move; you are ironing out the curve above it.

5 With your body moving in one piece – this time with a flat back – return to the sitting position in one smooth movement. Repeat the whole sequence four times.

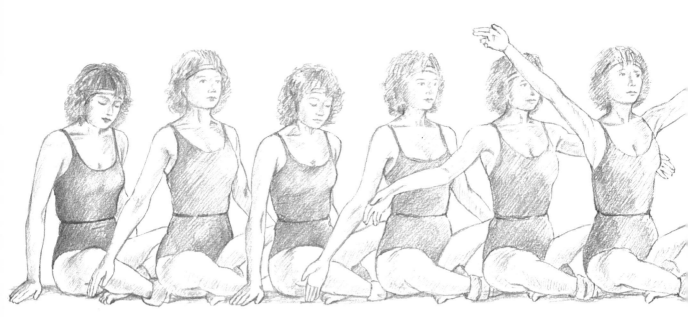

EXERCISE 65 ✱ ////////////////////

The last three exercises are contemporary dance movements called breathings. As the name suggests, you should feel as if your whole body breathes when you do them.

1 Sitting up straight, legs crossed, let the breath out and gently curve the whole spine, so that the small of your back is rounded and you are looking toward the floor. Your hands are on the floor in a straight line from your shoulders.

2 As you breathe in, grow tall through the spine, letting the air fill your whole body, the arms gently rounding out away from the body until only the fingertips are on the floor. The arms are moving from the middle of the back – not by lifting the shoulders. Eight times.

EXERCISE 66 ✱✱ ////////////////////

1 Start in the same position as the one you took up for the last exercise and breathe out, curving the spine.

2 This time, as you breathe in, take the movement through the arms and into the hands, so that they turn at the wrists and the palms face front. Breathe out and return to the starting position.

3 As you breathe in, extend the arms, lifting them off the ground, fingertips stretched. Check that your back is straight and not arching and that the arm movement is coming from the back, with your shoulders dropped and relaxed. Breathe out, drop the arms and curve the spine.

4 On this in-breath the arms reach up to a wide V-shape. Lower them as you breathe out and curve the back.

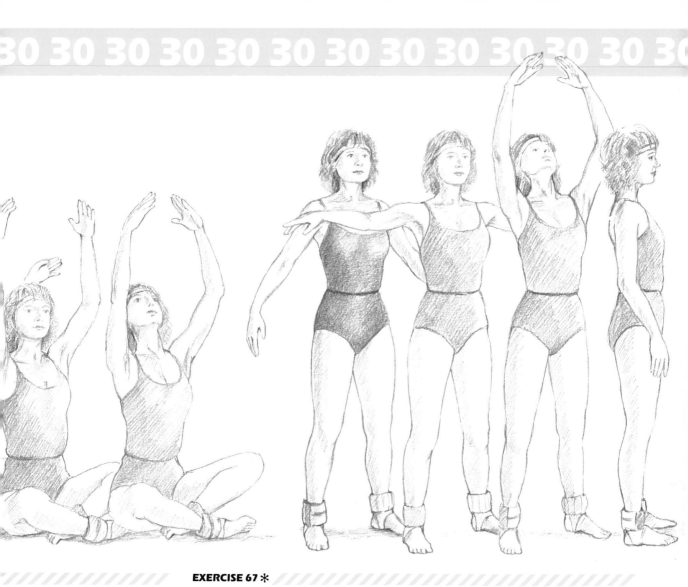

EXERCISE 67 ✳

5 This time, the in-breath takes the arms up and over the head. As you raise them, the arms should turn in the sockets, so that, at the top, the palms are facing each other. Lower the arms on the out-breath and curve the back.

6 On the last in-breath, take the movement up through the spine, so that you look into your hands. Your whole spine moves as well as your head, so that your upper chest is facing the ceiling as well. Breathe out as you lower the arms.

1 You start this last exercise standing straight, with your feet a hip width apart. Pull up your buttock and stomach muscles. Let your breath out. As you breathe in, let the air fill your body and lift your arms out gently to the side. Breathe out as you lower them.

2 On the next in-breath, take the arms up to shoulder height. Make sure that they are moving from the back and that they are really reaching right out through the fingertips. Breathe out and lower.

3 On the next in-breath, the arms come right up above the head, palms facing at the top. Breathe out and lower. Breathe in and take your arms up as before, but this time look into the hands, so mobilizing the whole of the upper spine as you did when sitting on the floor. Again, your chest, not just your face, reaches toward the ceiling.

4 Breathe out and bring your arms down to your sides. You should be standing up quite straight, your butt tucked under. Your knees, thighs and stomach muscles should be well pulled up, while your rib cage should feel full of air. The shoulders are dropped down into the back and relaxed. The head is proud and in line with the spine. You should now feel full of oxygen, totally energized and ready for anything!

71

Note: It is important when exercising weights that you proceed carefully to avoid injuring yourself. If you have not been exercising regularly, start the exercises without wearing weights. If you have problems with your back or any joints, be especially cautious. And exercise particular care during any exercise in which the arms or legs are extended away from the body. At the first sign of strain during any exercise, STOP. Consult your physician before continuing with the program.

Body Exercise

Once you have worked through the 30-minute routine with weights, you are ready to start working on the specific areas of the body that require individual attention to ensure that they are toned to peak perfection. The exercises here are designed to help you in this.

Follow the same basic rules as before. Work through the exercises without weights first and only add them when you feel your body is ready for them. If you feel any strain. stop and omit the exercise concerned until later in your program. And don't forget to unwind at the end of your work-out by working through the relaxation sequences as well.

Throughout the program, pay particular attention to your breathing, since correct breathing is just as important as the exercises themselves. What you should be aiming for is deep, regular breathing, paced to suit the specific movement. If you are doing a long stretch, for instance, you breathe in through your nose before starting the stretch and then breathe out slowly as you make the necessary physical effort to execute the stretch. Don't be tempted to hold your breath – this is counterproductive – and do not pant. Panting is a sign of strain, so if you find yourself doing this, it means that the exercise is too much for you.

THE UPPER BODY

The exercises in this section and the ones in the following three sections have been devised as extras to work on specific problem areas – many women, for instance, have flabby upper arms, which need special attention. They can also be used as substitutes for the relevant exercises in the Basic Routine. It is always a good idea to vary your exercises, as this will ensure they remain fun to do.

The upper body, particularly the neck and shoulders, is usually the main seat of tension. So this first section contains fuller versions of the neck rolls and shoulder circles in the Basic Routine to help you beat the problem. If you feel tension creeping in at any time, do one of these exercises, or simply let the head drop forward, chin toward the chest.

Never let the shoulders hunch up with tension; you should always have a mental image of lengthening the spine and stretching the arms to their fullest extension right through to the finger tips. In fact, throughout your exercising, keep the feeling of elongation in straight, clean lines, with a lifted head on a long neck.

The arms should always move from the center of the back and not from the shoulders. There should be space, too, between the ribs – don't let the body slump – and the chest should always feel open with dropped shoulders.

The "bosom-firmers" actually work on the pectoral muscles – the muscles behind the breasts. Good posture is vital, so think tall and don't forget to put energy into your movements.

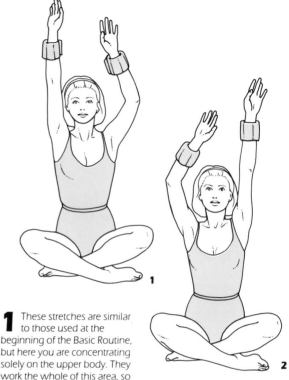

1 These stretches are similar to those used at the beginning of the Basic Routine, but here you are concentrating solely on the upper body. They work the whole of this area, so you should feel you are working right down the side and into the waist, not just the arm. Work through them quite slowly, really reaching out from the waist. You should sit on the floor and have weights attached to your wrists, **1**. Feel the arms working from the middle of the back and keep the shoulders dropped down. The whole body should lengthen out, **2**. 16 stretches, alternating.

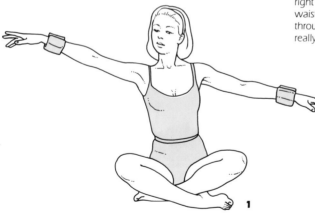

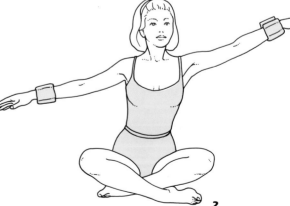

2 The side stretches lengthen the body in the same way as the upward ones. Don't slump into the waist and simply reach outwards. What you should do is to reach upwards first with the body, so that the ribs carry out to the side in one piece, **1**. Again, really stretch the arm right through to the fingertips, working it, as always, from the center of the back with a dropped shoulder, **2**.

As in the first exercise, take this very slowly and thoroughly. 16 stretches, alternating.

3 This is good for the flabby upper arms and for the pectorals. The arms are stretched out in front of you, crossed at the wrists, **1**. Starting low, cross them so that each time the alternate hand is on top, taking them higher each time. For this exercise to work, the arms should be fully extended right out through the fingertips, **2**.

Get to the top in eight cross-overs, **3**, and then repeat the crossing on the way down, making sure that your whole body is well lifted throughout and your head is in line with your spine. Don't look up at the ceiling when you get to the top, just keep looking straight ahead.

Do the whole exercise two to four times.

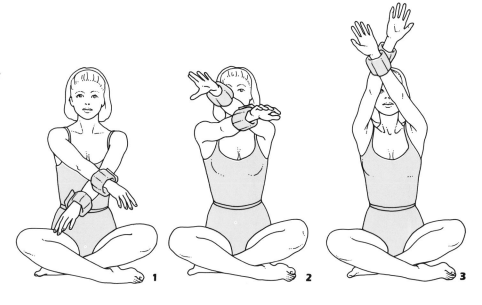

4 This exercise looks deceptively easy – in fact, it is a killer! There is nothing like it, though, for toning up the hands and the arms.

With the body well lifted out of the waist, have the arms stretched out low at the sides of the body, **1**. Clench the hands into fists, fling the fingers out hard, stretching them as far as they will go, **2**.

Now make a fist again, raising the arms a little as you do so. Fling out the fingers in the same way, **3**. Repeat in a smooth

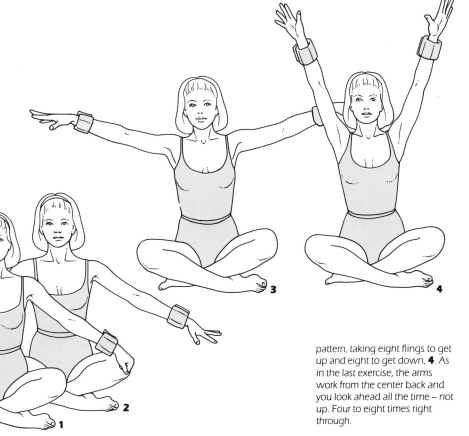

pattern, taking eight flings to get up and eight to get down, **4**. As in the last exercise, the arms work from the center back and you look ahead all the time – not up. Four to eight times right through.

5 This is another great exercise for the upper arm. Stretch upwards, **1**, reaching out of the waist, with the upper arm right next to the face. The palm is facing front and the stretch goes out through the fingertips,

Keeping the upper arm exactly where it is, hinge at the elbow, so that the forearm drops in a semi-circle behind the head, and gets as close in line with the upper arm as it can, **2**. Then retrace the semi-circle until the arm is vertical again, **3**.

Do this exercise slowly so that you can feel the arm muscles working. And it is very important to keep the back straight – don't arch. If you feel the effects in the back instead of the arm, stop. Four on each side.

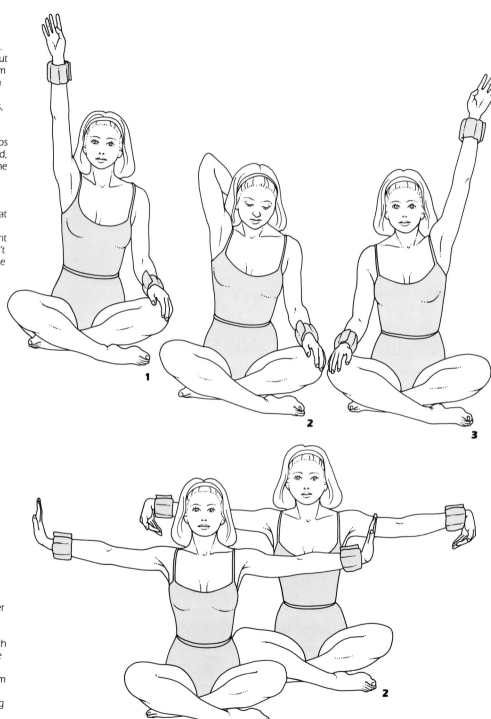

1

2

3

6 Another really effective assault on flabby upper arms! Sit with the arms fully extended to the side at shoulder level. Now flex the hands back hard, keeping the fingers straight, so that you feel a stretch right along the underside of the arm, **1**.

Drop the hands and curl them under as far as they will go, **2**. You should feel a real pull along the backs of the hands, wrists and forearms. Flex and drop 16 times.

1

2

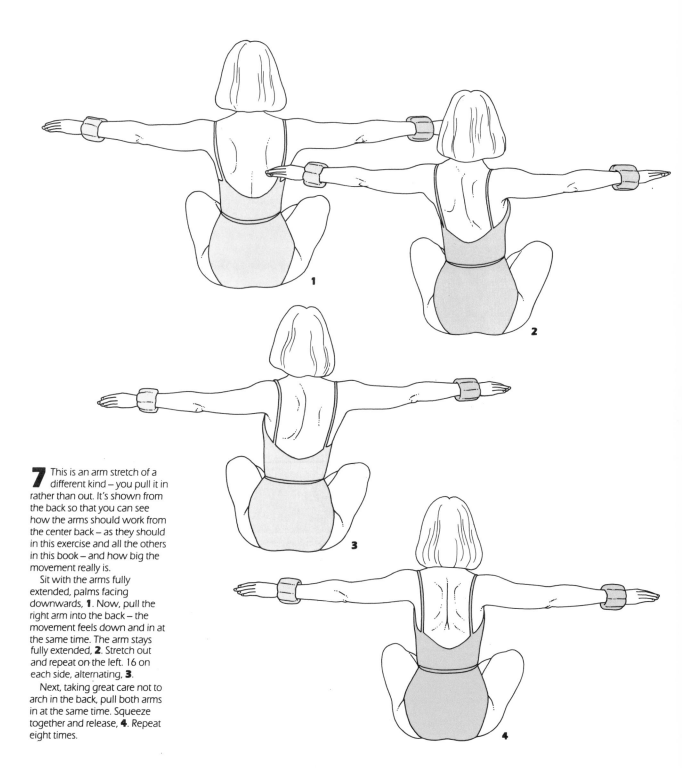

7 This is an arm stretch of a different kind – you pull it in rather than out. It's shown from the back so that you can see how the arms should work from the center back – as they should in this exercise and all the others in this book – and how big the movement really is.

Sit with the arms fully extended, palms facing downwards, **1**. Now, pull the right arm into the back – the movement feels down and in at the same time. The arm stays fully extended, **2**. Stretch out and repeat on the left. 16 on each side, alternating, **3**.

Next, taking great care not to arch in the back, pull both arms in at the same time. Squeeze together and release, **4**. Repeat eight times.

8 These shoulder exercises are a fuller version of the exercise in the Basic Routine, but now the weights are on the wrists, mainly as a reminder to lengthen the arms out fully. Keep the movement smooth and don't jerk it.

Start by lifting the shoulders up to the ears and letting them drop down again as you do in the routine, **1**. Eight times.

Now take them forwards and back. When they go back, the shoulder blades squeeze together, **2-3**. Eight times. Make a circle by taking the shoulders forwards, up, back and down. Remember that this is a smooth movement, **4-5**. Eight times.

The last part of the exercise is the shoulder circle which you do just as before, except now the hands rest on the shoulders, so that your elbows trace circles in the air, **6-8**. Eight times. If you feel any tension in the neck during this, drop the head forward on to the chest. If this doesn't help, stop. This is a marvelous way of loosening up the whole area of the back, neck and shoulders. Try the whole sequence through twice.

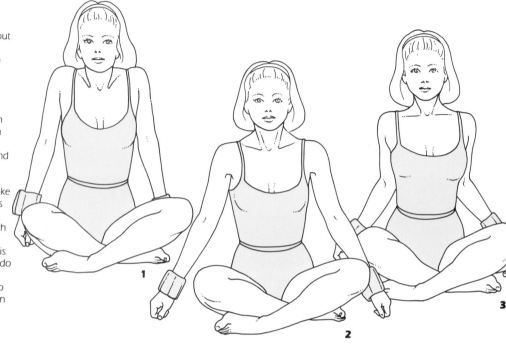

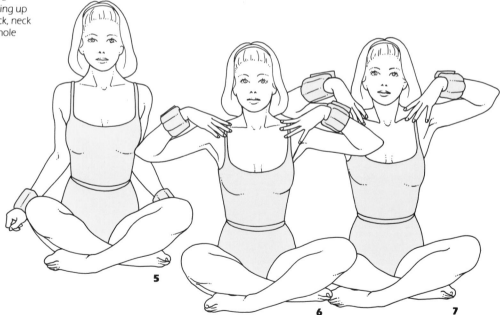

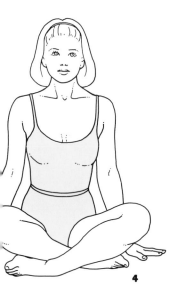

9 This is a good exercise for the neck and throat (which often get forgotten) and deals very effectively with double chins and sagging jaw lines. It uses the head as the weight, the hands just resting on the knees throughout. Sit up with a straight back, the head in line with a tall spine, **1**.

Drop your head back as far as it will go, so that you are looking up at the ceiling. You should feel the stretch up through the throat, **2**.

Now let the lower jaw drop so that your mouth is wide open, **3**. Then slowly close your mouth so that the bottom teeth are touching the top ones. This will increase the stretch considerably.

Raise the head so that you are looking straight ahead again, **4**. Eight times.

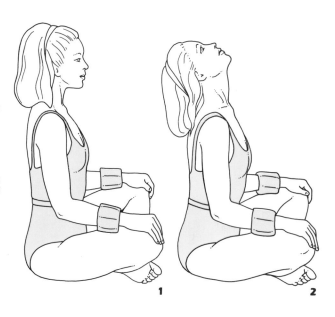

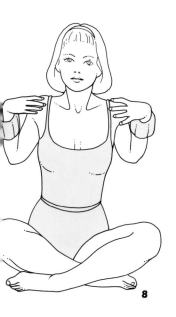

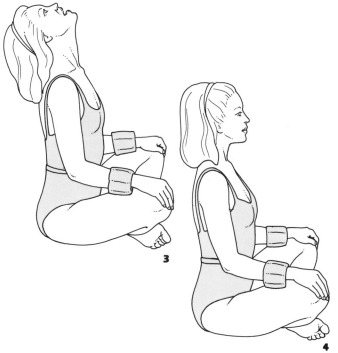

10 Though this exercise is mainly for loosening up the upper spine, it works the stomach as well. Lie flat on the floor, your legs stretched out and feet pointed, **1**.

Flex the feet and, at the same time, roll up as far as you can to look at them, **2**. Keep the chin on the chest and don't try to get much more than your middle back off the ground, as this is not a sit up. Eight times.

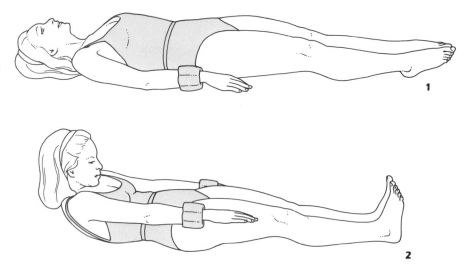

11 This is the full version of the neck rolls (the shorter variation is given on p. 34). Try this one only when you are sure that your neck and shoulders are supple enough for it. Again, it is the head which acts as the weight.

Start by looking straight in front of you, **1**. Then, turn the head to look as far as you can over your right shoulder, keeping the rest of your body still, **2**. You should feel a good stretch along the left side of the neck.

With your head in the same alignment, turn through the center, so that you are looking over the left shoulder, **3**. Eight times, alternating.

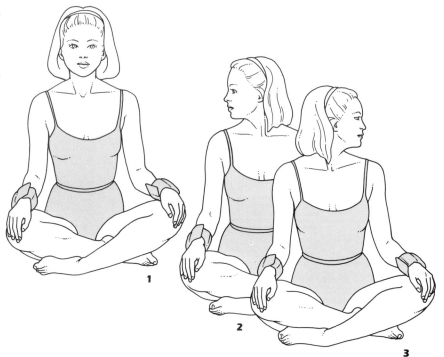

12 From the center position, drop your head straight back as far as it will go so that you are looking at the ceiling. Come back through the center, and drop the head down, so that the chin is on the chest, **1**. Eight times, alternating, feeling the stretch up the front of the throat as the head goes back and in the curve of the neck and upper back as the head drops forward.

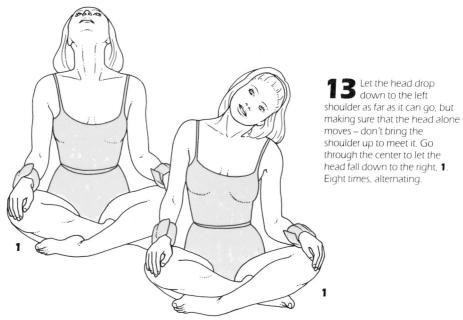

13 Let the head drop down to the left shoulder as far as it can go, but making sure that the head alone moves – don't bring the shoulder up to meet it. Go through the center to let the head fall down to the right, **1**. Eight times, alternating.

14 Now, taking the head in a tilt to the right, let it describe a half-circle forwards, **1**, through center and up to a tilt on the left, **2**. The head should feel very heavy and its weight should extend the neck. Repeat the half-circle starting on the left, **3**. Four half-circles.

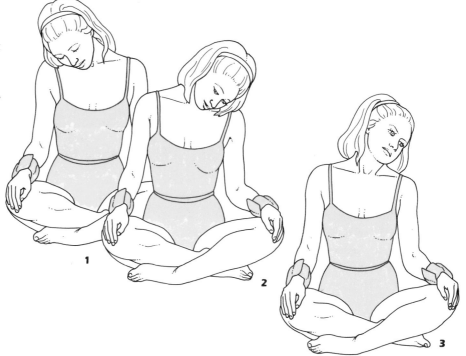

15 The final stage of this exercise is a full circle. Do not follow the entire sequence if you have back or shoulder problems, or are still stiff. If this is the case, just take the half-circles to the front. Again, begin by dropping the head in a tilt to the right and let it roll slowly forward across the chest to the left, **1, 2**. Instead of lifting the head back up to the center from a tilt on the left, let it continue to roll round in a circle to the back, **3**. Come back over the right shoulder to the center, **4**, raise the head and repeat the whole exercise, starting on the left.

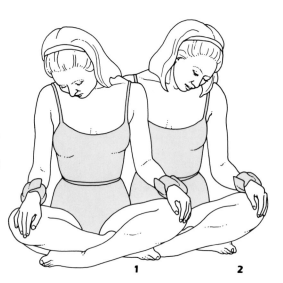
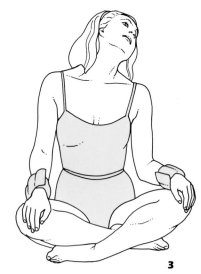

1   2   3

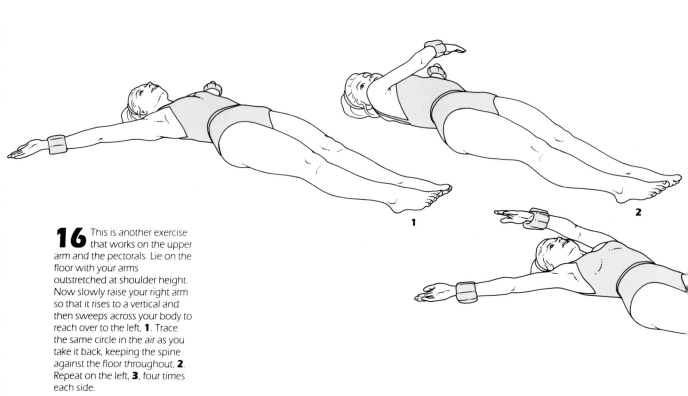

1   2

16 This is another exercise that works on the upper arm and the pectorals. Lie on the floor with your arms outstretched at shoulder height. Now slowly raise your right arm so that it rises to a vertical and then sweeps across your body to reach over to the left, **1**. Trace the same circle in the air as you take it back, keeping the spine against the floor throughout, **2**. Repeat on the left, **3**, four times each side.

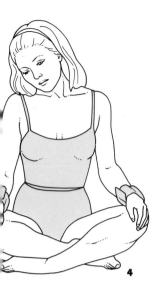

17 This is a particularly good bosom-firmer – it works on the pectorals, which are the muscles behind the breasts. Stretch your arms out to the sides at shoulder level, **1**. Now raise them above the head, so that the palms meet, making sure that the movement comes from the back and that the shoulders are dropped, **2**.

Start to lower the hands, pressing them hard together as you do so. If you are doing this correctly, you should feel the pectorals working straight away – it should almost feel as if it is the pectorals that are pulling the arms down. Lower the arms until the hands are in line with the breast bone, **3**. You will feel the upper arm muscles working as well. Four times.

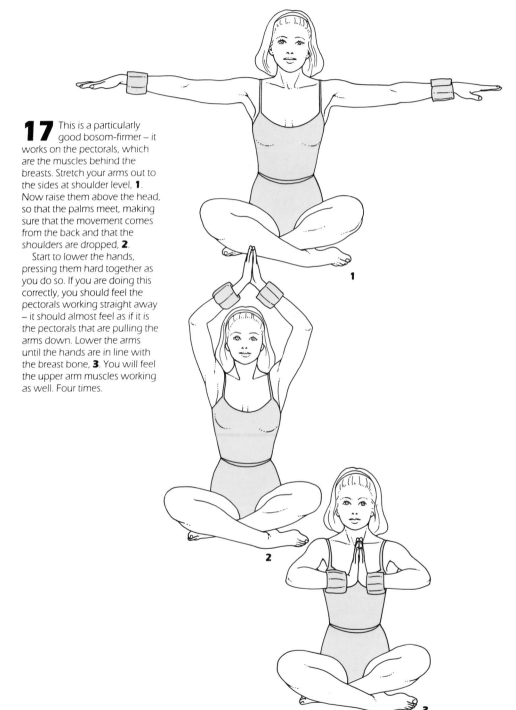

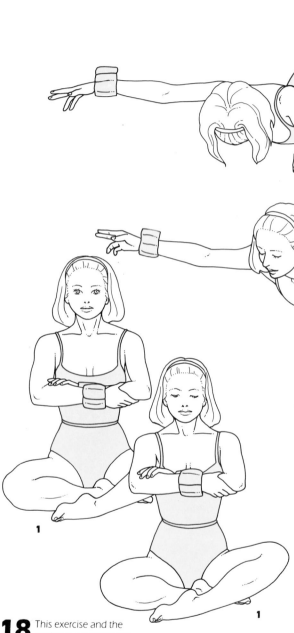

21 This last long exercise is a contemporary dance movement; the complete sequence is a complex one to learn. The spiraling in the hip socket is a small movement as well as one that is difficult to locate, so make sure that you have located the spiral exactly before you start to string all the elements of the sequence together. The upper body is involved – especially in the later part of the sequence – but the initial, vital movement comes from the hip socket.

Sit on the floor, weights on the ankles, crossed-legged, right foot in front, **1**. Make sure that you are well up on your sitting bones – that means holding the buttocks firm. Your arms should be relaxed but extended fully, so that your wrists are resting on your knees, the hand pointing out beyond them. The upper part of the body is held well up, but, if you relax, it will follow the hip movement, not lead the way. If you find it difficult to locate the spiral in the hip, try it with your legs straight out in front of you, hand on hip.

Pull back the right hip; if anything the movement is an upward one, so don't drop down. **2**. Don't try to make this a big movement – it isn't. If you are doing it correctly, however, you will feel "echoes" throughout the body. You will find that you will turn slightly above the hip toward the right and your left hand will now be out in front of the right, **3**. You should not make a conscious effort to anticipate these movements; they will happen naturally as you spiral.

Return to the center, **4**, and repeat, this time pulling back the left hip, **5**. Try four on each side to really get the feel of the movement before you extend it into the next stage of the sequence.

In this, you let the head follow the turning of the spine. So, when you pull back the right hip, the body spirals toward the

20 This exercise can follow on from the series of stretches in the Basic Routine. It is an exercise for the legs and buttocks as much as for the upper body.

Lie on the floor, face down, the weights on the ankles, or wrists, or both, depending on your strength. Raise the head and the chest up from the floor at the same time as the legs. Only the ribs and hips should still be in contact with the floor, **1**.

Stretch the arms out to the sides, feeling the chest very open, head in line with the spine and neck open and relaxed. There should be no tension in the neck or shoulders. Now, holding the buttock muscles very hard, tap the feet together, **2**. 50 times.

18 This exercise and the next one are two more good bosom-firmers.

Clasp the arms at the elbows with the opposite hands. Without tensing up the shoulders, try to pull the arms away from each other – but not letting go. Pull and release eight times, **1**.

19 The next stage is simply the reverse of the previous one. Instead of pulling the arms apart, push and release eight times, taking care that it is the pectorals and not the neck and shoulders, that are doing the work, **1**.

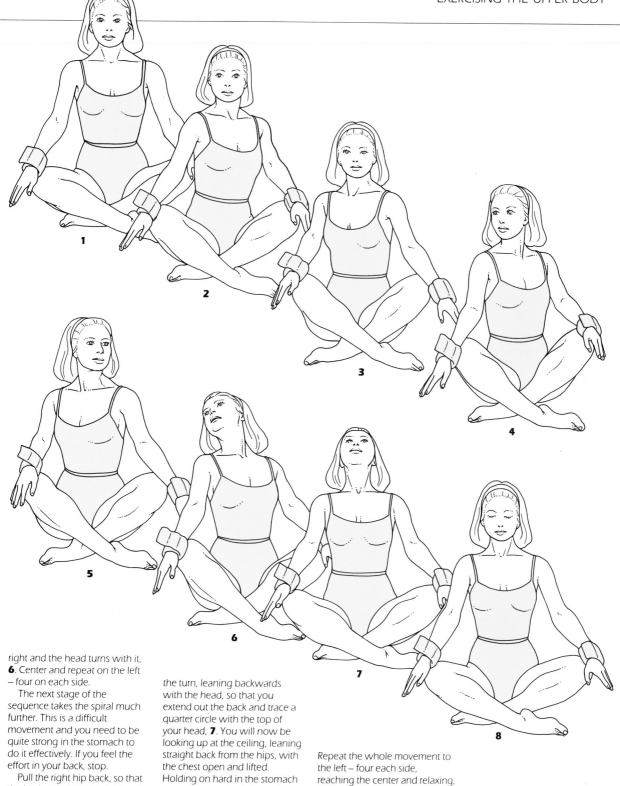

right and the head turns with it, **6**. Center and repeat on the left – four on each side.

The next stage of the sequence takes the spiral much further. This is a difficult movement and you need to be quite strong in the stomach to do it effectively. If you feel the effort in your back, stop.

Pull the right hip back, so that the body spirals to the right and the head turns. Now exaggerate the turn, leaning backwards with the head, so that you extend out the back and trace a quarter circle with the top of your head, **7**. You will now be looking up at the ceiling, leaning straight back from the hips, with the chest open and lifted. Holding on hard in the stomach muscles, come back "over the top" to the center and relax, **8**.

Repeat the whole movement to the left – four each side, reaching the center and relaxing, letting the breath right out each time you return to the center.

WAIST AND STOMACH

The stomach muscles are often some of the weakest ones in a woman's body. It is a common fault to try to make up for this weakness by letting the back take the strain. This should be avoided at all costs, as you can really hurt your back in this way. So, if your stomach muscles start to bulge or quiver at any time, you are attempting something which is beyond them. Try an easier exercise or do the same thing but without weights. Always remember; too, that if you are lying on your back, the lower your legs are toward the floor, the more strain you will be putting on the stomach muscles.

The main point to remember here is never to let the small of your back arch to take the strain. Always keep the navel lifted up and back as if it is trying to press itself against the spine.

The feeling you are aiming for here, as always, is that of elongation. Keep the spine straight, the tailbone dropping straight down toward the floor, and stretch the body up out of the waist.

The contraction is one of the most important elements in working this area and is described in detail on page 64 and in the exercises which use it on page 64-67. When you "move in one piece" you should be aiming to keep your contraction held perfectly in place as you carry it forward or back into another spatial position.

Try to think in these exercises – and indeed all the time – of the stomach muscles providing a natural girdle, keeping the body in a lifted, well-held posture.

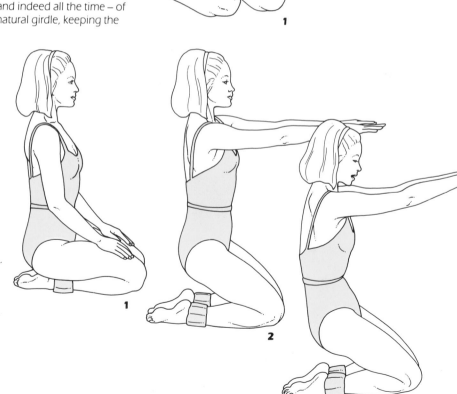

22 This is a good exercise for both the stomach and the buttocks. Kneel down, your hands resting on your knees, keeping your back straight. The maximum amount of lift should only be about a few inches, **1**.

Using the same contraction as you did in the Basic Routine (pp64-65), pull back hard as the navel presses against the back, curve slightly at the waist and pull the butt muscles under hard, **2**. Sit down and release.

Do this four times and then try reversing the movement, so that you start by coming up in a pelvic tilt, **3**. Release, straighten, and then sit back down. Four times.

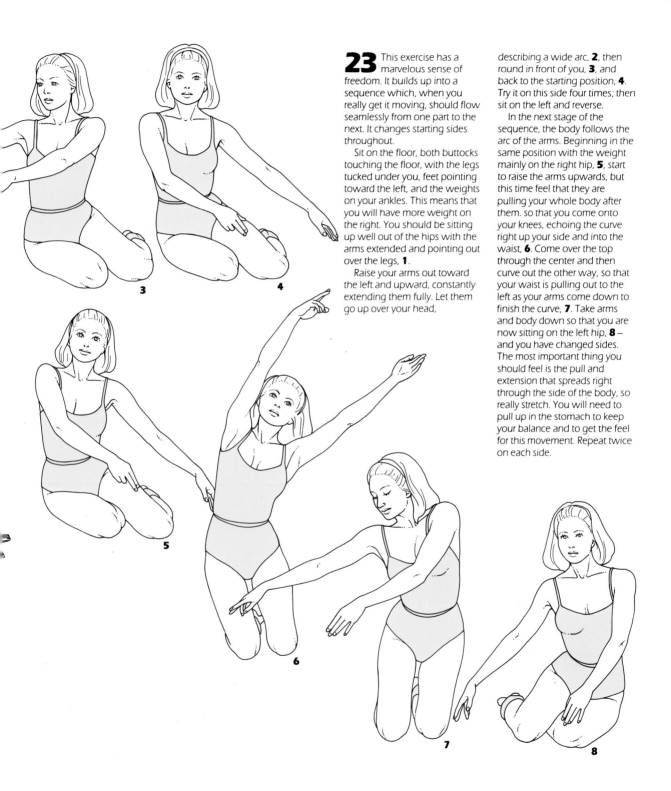

23 This exercise has a marvelous sense of freedom. It builds up into a sequence which, when you really get it moving, should flow seamlessly from one part to the next. It changes starting sides throughout.

Sit on the floor, both buttocks touching the floor, with the legs tucked under you, feet pointing toward the left, and the weights on your ankles. This means that you will have more weight on the right. You should be sitting up well out of the hips with the arms extended and pointing out over the legs, **1**.

Raise your arms out toward the left and upward, constantly extending them fully. Let them go up over your head, describing a wide arc, **2**, then round in front of you, **3**, and back to the starting position, **4**. Try it on this side four times; then sit on the left and reverse.

In the next stage of the sequence, the body follows the arc of the arms. Beginning in the same position with the weight mainly on the right hip, **5**, start to raise the arms upwards, but this time feel that they are pulling your whole body after them. so that you come onto your knees, echoing the curve right up your side and into the waist, **6**. Come over the top through the center and then curve out the other way, so that your waist is pulling out to the left as your arms come down to finish the curve, **7**. Take arms and body down so that you are now sitting on the left hip, **8** – and you have changed sides. The most important thing you should feel is the pull and extension that spreads right through the side of the body, so really stretch. You will need to pull up in the stomach to keep your balance and to get the feel for this movement. Repeat twice on each side.

Start as before, sitting on the left hip, **9**, and come up in a long curve, bending at the waist toward the left, **10**. Come over the top and curve the body out to the right, body and arms making a wide, open semi-circle, **11**.

Come down as if to sit on the right hip, but, instead of sitting, let the arms complete the circle in front of the body, **12**. Use them as a balance on the floor as you start to take the whole of your right side down to lie on the floor, **13**. As your side starts to reach the floor, your top (left) leg starts to rise. so that, by the time your body is flat, your leg is high in the air, extended right out, toes pointed, **14**. Your bottom (right) leg is bent underneath you for support. Take your top leg over as far as you can, and then lower it as you raise your body up from the ground, **15**.

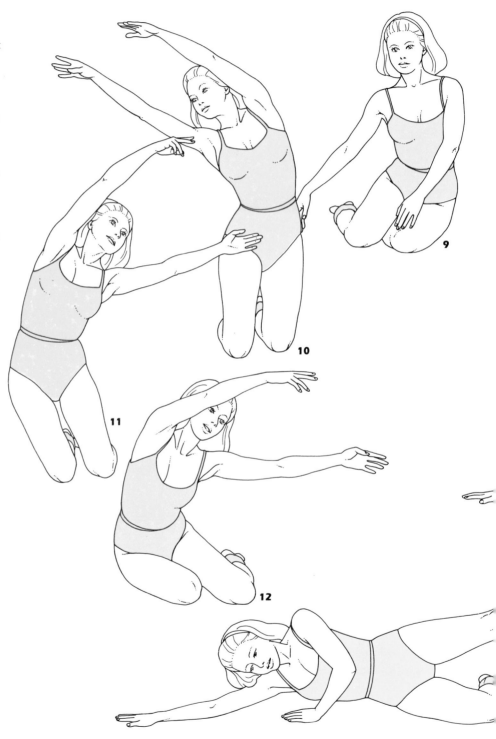

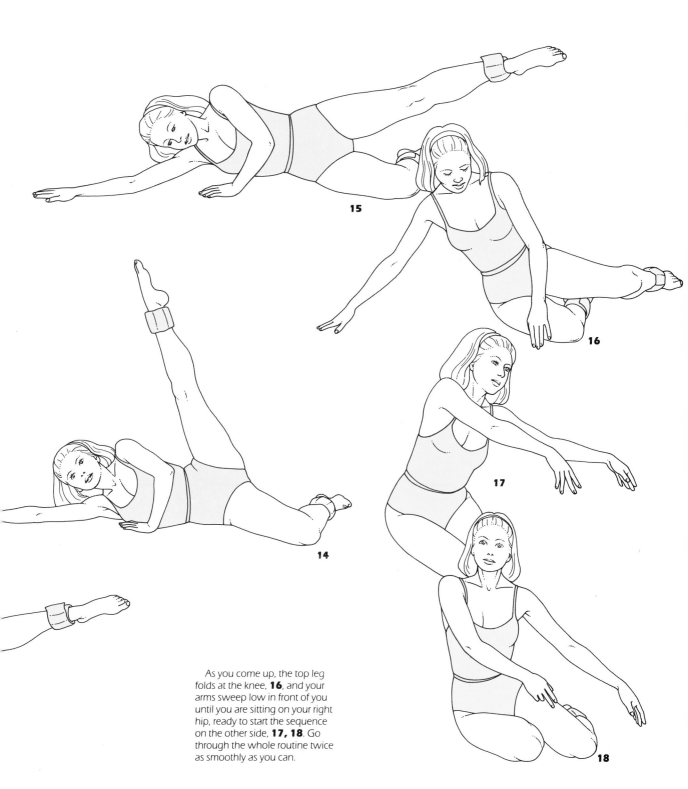

As you come up, the top leg folds at the knee, **16**, and your arms sweep low in front of you until you are sitting on your right hip, ready to start the sequence on the other side, **17, 18**. Go through the whole routine twice as smoothly as you can.

24 This is a good exercise for the stomach and butt, too. The important thing to remember is that the stomach is doing all the work of lifting the leg. As always, should you feel that your back is straining, stop and try a more gentle stomach exercise until the muscles get stronger.

Lie flat on the floor, the arms stretched out at shoulder height, stomach and butt muscles held in, **1**. Start to retrace a circle with your right foot, keeping your leg on the floor.

Inevitably, you will soon have to lift the leg from the floor, but keep it as low as you can, **2**. Take it up as far as possible, until you have to turn it inwards to come over your body, **3**.

Now take it over, so that it crosses your body and continues to trace the same wide circle, **4**. You will probably find at this point that your back comes off the floor so that you are leaning over to the left. Try to avoid this, as it is important to keep the body still throughout; just let the leg do the traveling, held by the stomach muscles.

Continue the circle until the moving leg has crossed the other to return to the starting position, **5**. Repeat the exercise twice on each side.

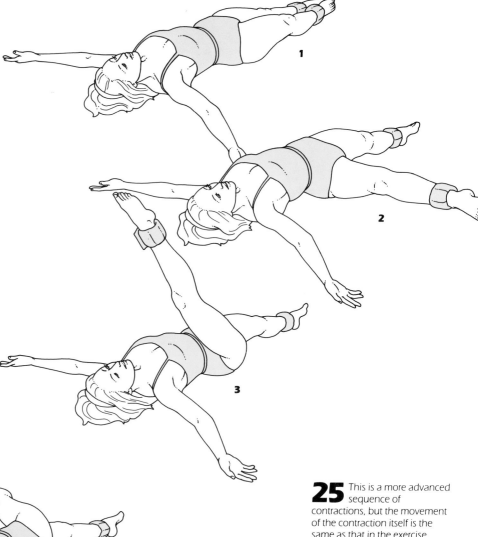

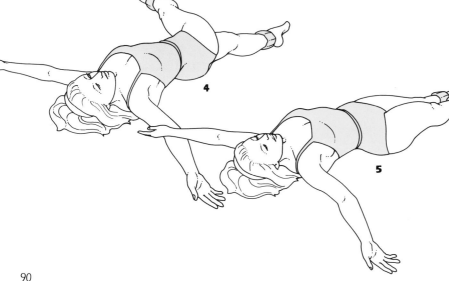

25 This is a more advanced sequence of contractions, but the movement of the contraction itself is the same as that in the exercise shown in the Basic Routine on page 39. The difference is that now you follow it through in three different positions.

The first position is the closest to the one shown in the Basic Routine, but now, instead of having the legs crossed, you sit with the soles of the feet together. You should be sitting very tall with a straight back, the arms and chest open, the hands on the ankles, **1**

Contract, scooping out in the stomach, gently rounding the back and pulling the butt under you in a pelvic tilt. The chest and shoulders are soft – don't tense them, **2**.

Take the contraction forward in one piece, so that the head reaches down toward the ankles, **3**. However, the body retains exactly the same shape as it did when in the upright stage of the original contraction. Release the contraction, without changing the position of the hips, so that the back straightens out in a strong, flat diagonal stretch. You will feel this movement open out the thighs. Don't round the back to get lower – it is the straightness of the back that counts, **4**.

Return to the starting position by lifting, again in one controlled movement, without shifting the hips. After this, check that you are lifted throughout the whole body, high on the sitting bones and without any stiffness in the neck or shoulders. You will only have managed this if you have really been using the stomach. Repeat four times.

26 The next exercise is a continuation of the last one, but now the contraction is taken in a different position. Sit with the front legs pointed frontways straight out in front of you, the body well lifted out of the hips, **1**.

As you contract, pull back as though someone has grabbed you by the waist. You should not curve over, but there should be a strong feeling of being pulled in two directions at once, the body reaching away from the arms and legs. Flex both the hands and the feet and let the curve continue through the spine so that you look toward your feet, **2**.

Keeping the hips still, release the contraction, reaching

forward as before with a flat back and a long, straight diagonal, **3**. Don't forget that your head is part of your spine and should be in the same diagonal line, not looking up. This part of the sequence involves just as much hard work as any other – really feel stretched as if someone is pulling you by your arms in a long straight line from the hips.

Return to the starting position and repeat four times.

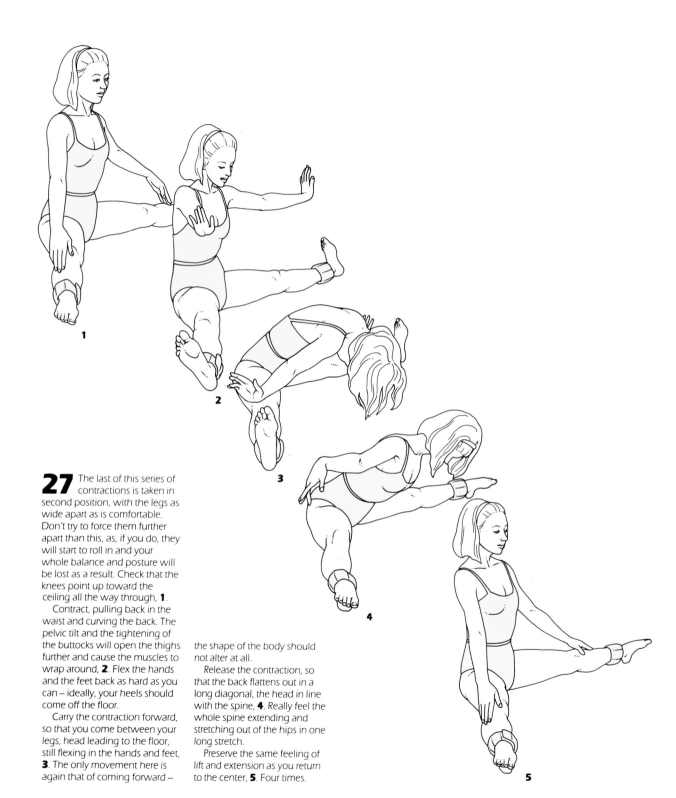

27 The last of this series of contractions is taken in second position, with the legs as wide apart as is comfortable. Don't try to force them further apart than this, as, if you do, they will start to roll in and your whole balance and posture will be lost as a result. Check that the knees point up toward the ceiling all the way through, **1**.

Contract, pulling back in the waist and curving the back. The pelvic tilt and the tightening of the buttocks will open the thighs further and cause the muscles to wrap around, **2**. Flex the hands and the feet back as hard as you can – ideally, your heels should come off the floor.

Carry the contraction forward, so that you come between your legs, head leading to the floor, still flexing in the hands and feet, **3**. The only movement here is again that of coming forward –

the shape of the body should not alter at all.

Release the contraction, so that the back flattens out in a long diagonal, the head in line with the spine, **4**. Really feel the whole spine extending and stretching out of the hips in one long stretch.

Preserve the same feeling of lift and extension as you return to the center, **5**. Four times.

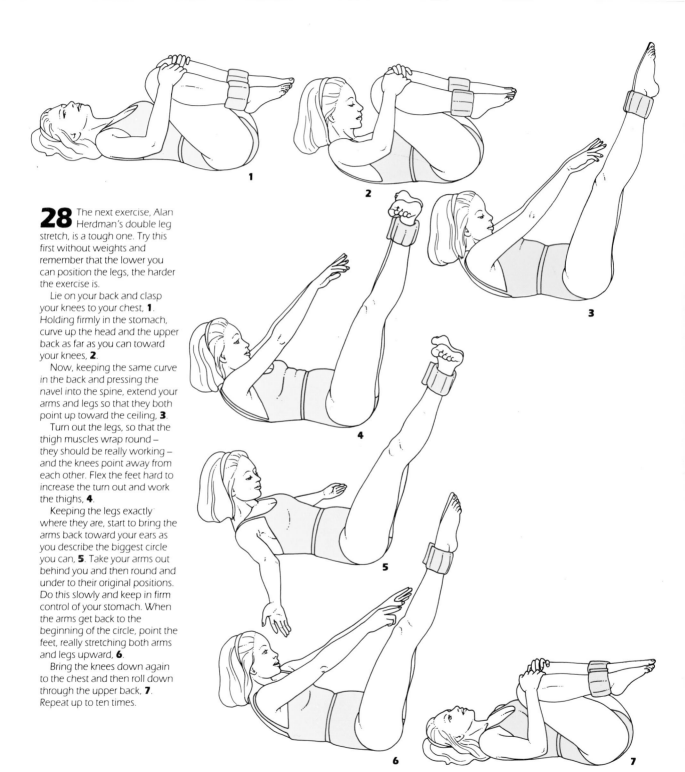

28 The next exercise, Alan Herdman's double leg stretch, is a tough one. Try this first without weights and remember that the lower you can position the legs, the harder the exercise is.

Lie on your back and clasp your knees to your chest, **1**. Holding firmly in the stomach, curve up the head and the upper back as far as you can toward your knees, **2**.

Now, keeping the same curve in the back and pressing the navel into the spine, extend your arms and legs so that they both point up toward the ceiling, **3**.

Turn out the legs, so that the thigh muscles wrap round – they should be really working – and the knees point away from each other. Flex the feet hard to increase the turn out and work the thighs, **4**.

Keeping the legs exactly where they are, start to bring the arms back toward your ears as you describe the biggest circle you can, **5**. Take your arms out behind you and then round and under to their original positions. Do this slowly and keep in firm control of your stomach. When the arms get back to the beginning of the circle, point the feet, really stretching both arms and legs upward, **6**.

Bring the knees down again to the chest and then roll down through the upper back, **7**. Repeat up to ten times.

29 For these waist twists, it is important to remember that it is only the waist and upper body which are turning – the hips stay absolutely still and facing the front. With weights on the wrists stand with the feet a hip width apart, the feet slightly turned out and the knees bent. The hands rest lightly on the shoulders, the arms well lifted. There should be no arching in the back, the tailbone dropping straight down toward the floor, **1**. Knees and hips facing front, turn from the waist to look over your right shoulder, **2**. 16 little turns, then repeat on the left, **3**.

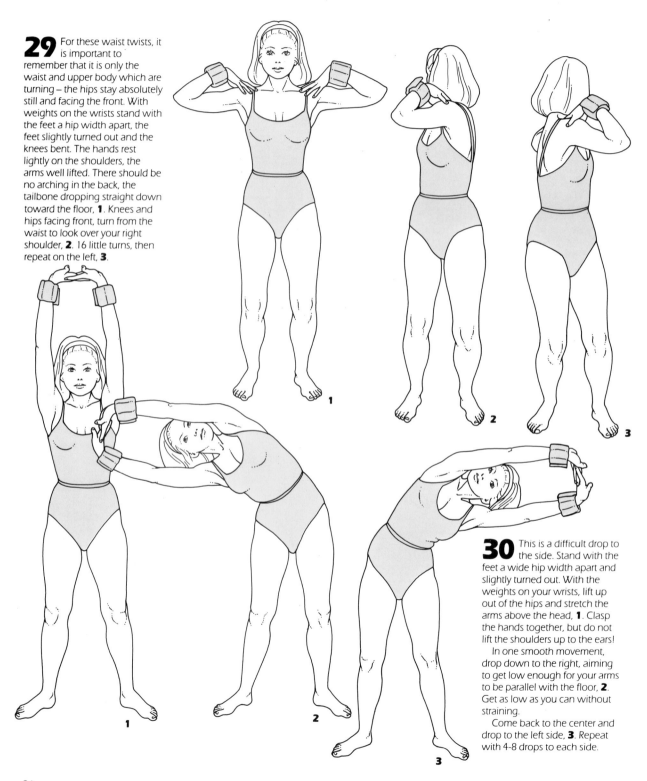

30 This is a difficult drop to the side. Stand with the feet a wide hip width apart and slightly turned out. With the weights on your wrists, lift up out of the hips and stretch the arms above the head, **1**. Clasp the hands together, but do not lift the shoulders up to the ears!

In one smooth movement, drop down to the right, aiming to get low enough for your arms to be parallel with the floor, **2**. Get as low as you can without straining.

Come back to the center and drop to the left side, **3**. Repeat with 4-8 drops to each side.

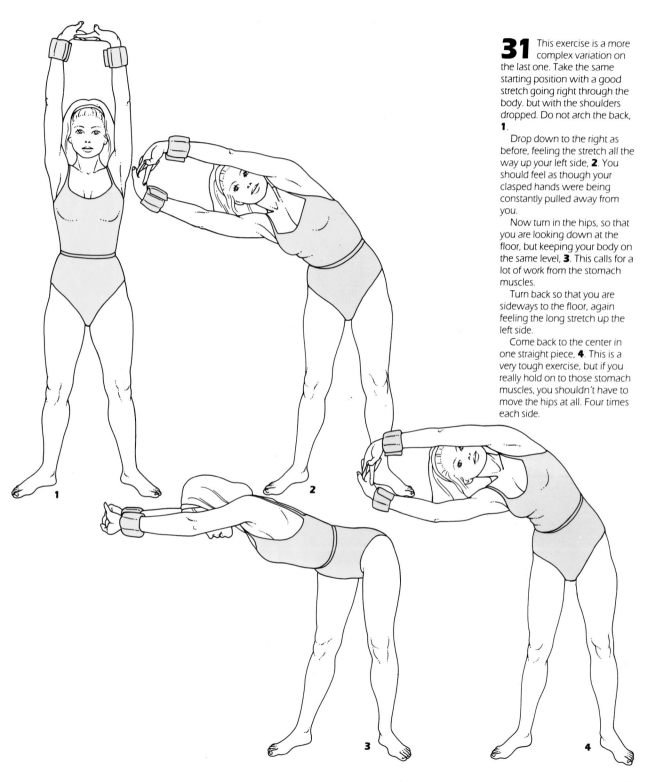

31 This exercise is a more complex variation on the last one. Take the same starting position with a good stretch going right through the body. but with the shoulders dropped. Do not arch the back, **1**.

Drop down to the right as before, feeling the stretch all the way up your left side, **2**. You should feel as though your clasped hands were being constantly pulled away from you.

Now turn in the hips, so that you are looking down at the floor, but keeping your body on the same level, **3**. This calls for a lot of work from the stomach muscles.

Turn back so that you are sideways to the floor, again feeling the long stretch up the left side.

Come back to the center in one straight piece, **4**. This is a very tough exercise, but if you really hold on to those stomach muscles, you shouldn't have to move the hips at all. Four times each side.

32 This is one of the most difficult of the waistline exercises, especially the back stretch, so add the weights only when you feel completely supple and proficient. Eventually the sequence should build up to 16 stretches on each side, followed by eight, four and two, and a circular sweep to the recovery position. Finish with a sweep incorporating the stretch to the back. Start with eight stretches to each side and build up gradually. The final stretch back is a lovely movement and feels wonderful, but it is difficult and only for those with strong and supple backs.

Keep the thighs and buttocks in contact with the ground – the weights are there to remind you to do this. The arms must always align with the body, never reach behind it.

Sit with your legs comfortably wide apart, toes pointed, **1**. Throughout, your knees should be pointing at the ceiling, never rolling inward. Always hold your back completely straight – this is important for posture.

Keeping your back straight, take your left arm up over your head and reach out along your right leg with your body at right angles to it, **2**. It does not matter how close your body is to your

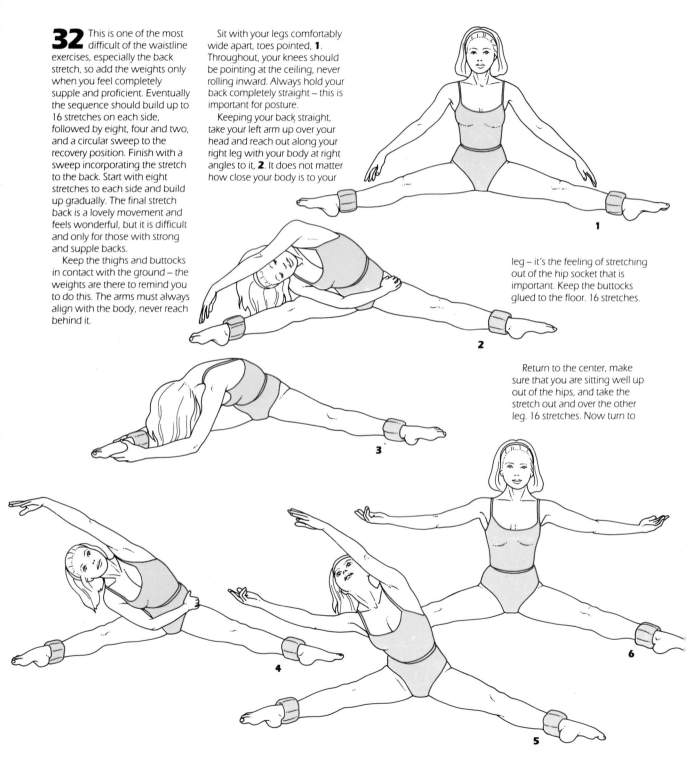

leg – it's the feeling of stretching out of the hip socket that is important. Keep the buttocks glued to the floor. 16 stretches.

Return to the center, make sure that you are sitting well up out of the hips, and take the stretch out and over the other leg. 16 stretches. Now turn to face your right leg and, holding the calf or the ankle (depending on how supple you are), lower yourself gently down toward your leg, **3**. Don't pull too hard and make sure that both hips are still in contact with the floor. 16 bounces.

Turn in the hip socket, so that you are facing front and stretching out sideways along the leg, trying to flatten out along it, **4**. Again don't force the movement. 16 stretches.

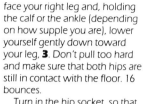

Come up so that you are in a diagonal line (at 45°) out of the side and really stretch out of the hip sockets for 16 stretches, **5**. Don't tense in the shoulders, or come off the floor.

Return to the center, **6**, and repeat the last three sets of 16 stretches to the left. Then, as you get stronger, repeat again for eight on each side, then on four and on two until you are ready for the long sweeping semi-circle which is the next part of the sequence.

The circle now goes forward between your legs, instead of in a vertical curve from side to side. Stretch out and to the side as before, **7**. leading down toward the right leg. As you get close to the leg, change the position of the body, so that you face down toward the floor, **8**.

Leading with the left arm, start to draw a wide arc across the floor, or in the air, depending on how supple you are.

Concentrate on keeping your back absolutely straight, correcting any over-arching, as this can be harmful. Check that your knees have not rolled inward and that your arms are stretching out from the middle of your back – no hunching!

As the left arm reaches the left leg, let it fall loosely across your waist and take the right arm over your head, **9**. Reach up and out of the hips, **10**, and stretch up from the floor until you are again sitting in the center, legs and feet fully extended and arms lifted to the sides with relaxed dropped shoulders. Stay in the center position, but flex the feet back as hard as you can – the movement is really working if the heels come off the floor, **11**.

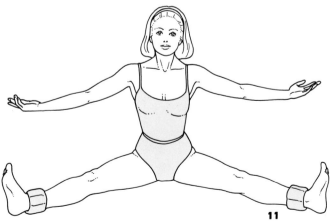

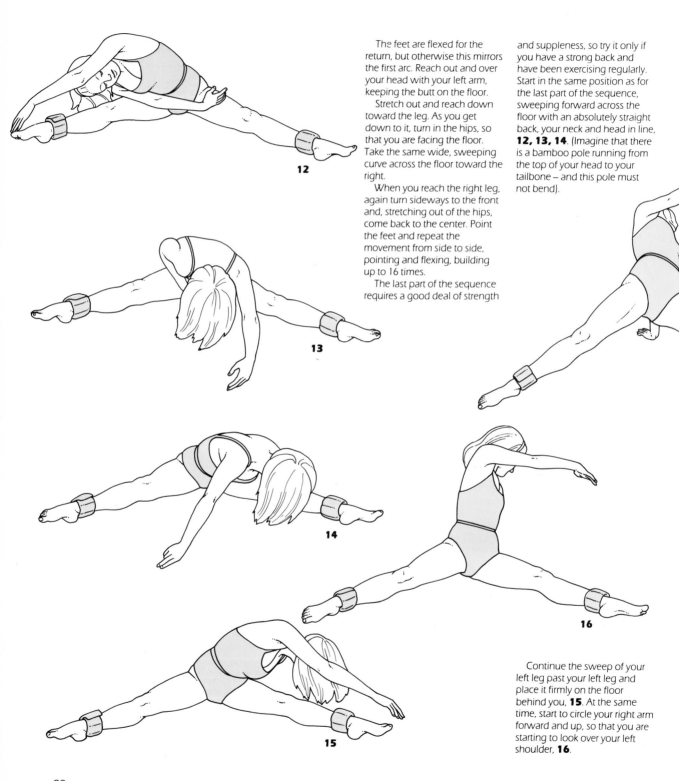

The feet are flexed for the return, but otherwise this mirrors the first arc. Reach out and over your head with your left arm, keeping the butt on the floor.

Stretch out and reach down toward the leg. As you get down to it, turn in the hips, so that you are facing the floor. Take the same wide, sweeping curve across the floor toward the right.

When you reach the right leg, again turn sideways to the front and, stretching out of the hips, come back to the center. Point the feet and repeat the movement from side to side, pointing and flexing, building up to 16 times.

The last part of the sequence requires a good deal of strength and suppleness, so try it only if you have a strong back and have been exercising regularly. Start in the same position as for the last part of the sequence, sweeping forward across the floor with an absolutely straight back, your neck and head in line, **12, 13, 14**. (Imagine that there is a bamboo pole running from the top of your head to your tailbone – and this pole must not bend).

12

13

14

15

16

Continue the sweep of your left leg past your left leg and place it firmly on the floor behind you, **15**. At the same time, start to circle your right arm forward and up, so that you are starting to look over your left shoulder, **16**.

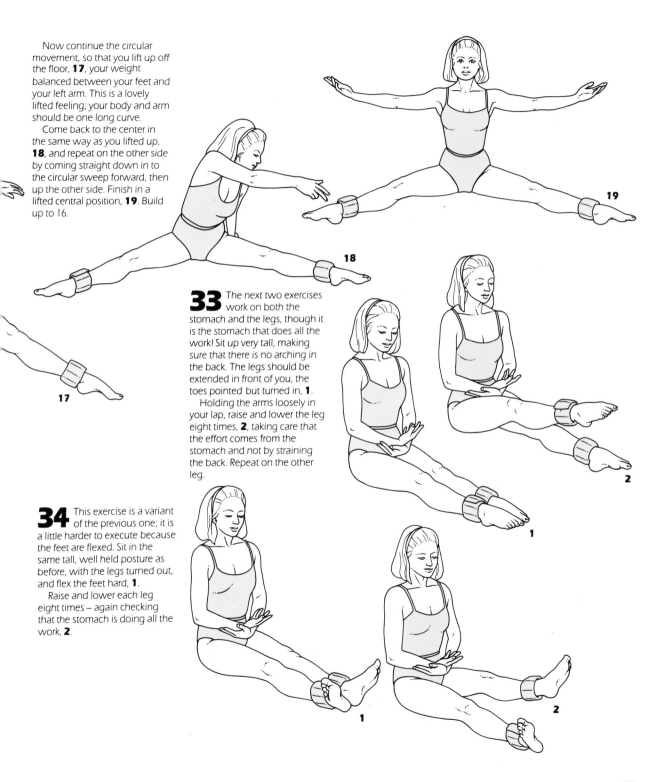

Now continue the circular movement, so that you lift up off the floor, **17**, your weight balanced between your feet and your left arm. This is a lovely lifted feeling; your body and arm should be one long curve.

Come back to the center in the same way as you lifted up, **18**, and repeat on the other side by coming straight down in to the circular sweep forward, then up the other side. Finish in a lifted central position, **19**. Build up to 16.

33 The next two exercises work on both the stomach and the legs, though it is the stomach that does all the work! Sit up very tall, making sure that there is no arching in the back. The legs should be extended in front of you, the toes pointed but turned in, **1**.

Holding the arms loosely in your lap, raise and lower the leg eight times, **2**, taking care that the effort comes from the stomach and not by straining the back. Repeat on the other leg.

34 This exercise is a variant of the previous one; it is a little harder to execute because the feet are flexed. Sit in the same tall, well held posture as before, with the legs turned out, and flex the feet hard, **1**.

Raise and lower each leg eight times – again checking that the stomach is doing all the work, **2**.

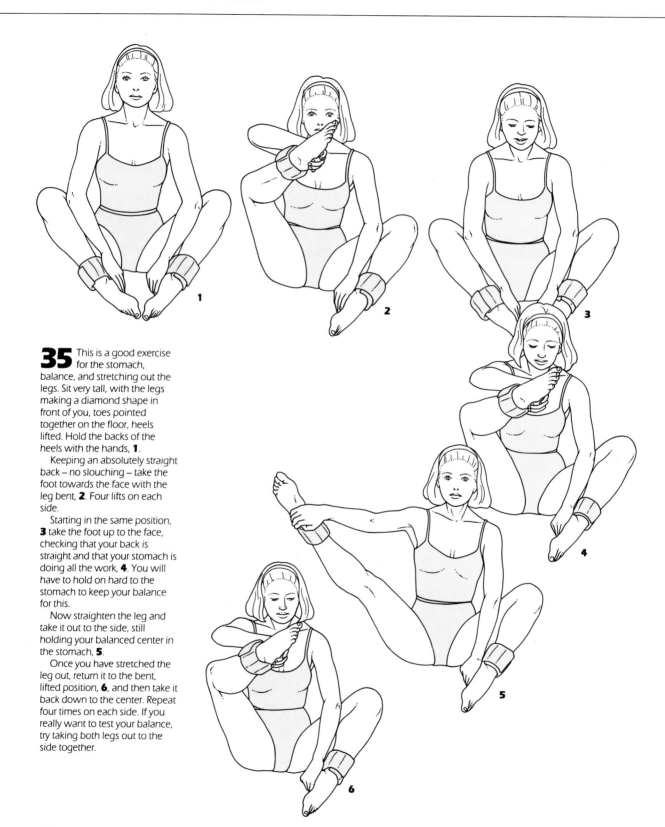

35 This is a good exercise for the stomach, balance, and stretching out the legs. Sit very tall, with the legs making a diamond shape in front of you, toes pointed together on the floor, heels lifted. Hold the backs of the heels with the hands, **1**.

Keeping an absolutely straight back – no slouching – take the foot towards the face with the leg bent, **2**. Four lifts on each side.

Starting in the same position, **3** take the foot up to the face, checking that your back is straight and that your stomach is doing all the work, **4**. You will have to hold on hard to the stomach to keep your balance for this.

Now straighten the leg and take it out to the side, still holding your balanced center in the stomach, **5**.

Once you have stretched the leg out, return it to the bent, lifted position, **6**, and then take it back down to the center. Repeat four times on each side. If you really want to test your balance, try taking both legs out to the side together.

BUTTOCKS AND LEGS

With the buttocks and legs, always remember to use them to their fullest extent – elongating the muscles to their fullest stretch with the knees pulled up and directly above the feet. The positions for the feet and legs are described on page 51.

When you lift your leg, the stretch should go right through its whole length and, if it is pointed, out through the toes too. If it is a flexed position, your heel should be flexed back hard and 'lead' the movement of the leg. There is a real difference between pointed and flexed feet so always make sure you can feel it and stretch them hard whichever way is required. Don't let the feet sickle – turn inward – keep them straight and in line or you will weaken the ankles.

"Turn out" is explained fully on page 51, but the essential thing to remember is that you turn the whole leg from the hip socket – your feet merely follow that movement as far as it will go. Never force your feet into a wider V-shape than the rest of your legs, or your knees will roll inward and you will lose your posture as well as courting danger for your knees and back.

Many of the exercises in this section use the stomach muscles too. Your legs weigh a lot, so they can impose a considerable strain on the stomach. If you feel yourself arching in the back, the exercise is too strong for you and you should try an easier one or take off the weights.

Lastly, if you are using a chairback for balance, remember to change sides halfway through each exercise so that each side is worked equally.

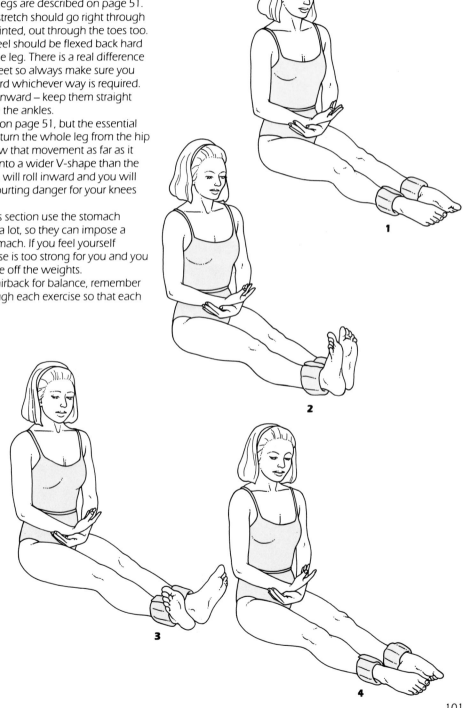

36 This is not only an excellent ankle exercise; it affects the rest of the leg as well. Sit up very tall – just because you are concentrating on the legs and feet, you shouldn't forget to keep your back straight and stomach pulled up.

With your feet parallel and pointed, flex back hard, **2**. With the feet still flexed, turn out, so that the thigh muscles wrap round and the butt tightens, **3**. You will probably grow an inch or two! Now, keeping the turn-out, point the feet, **4**. You will find that this is a very difficult stretch. Return to the parallel and repeat the sequence eight times.

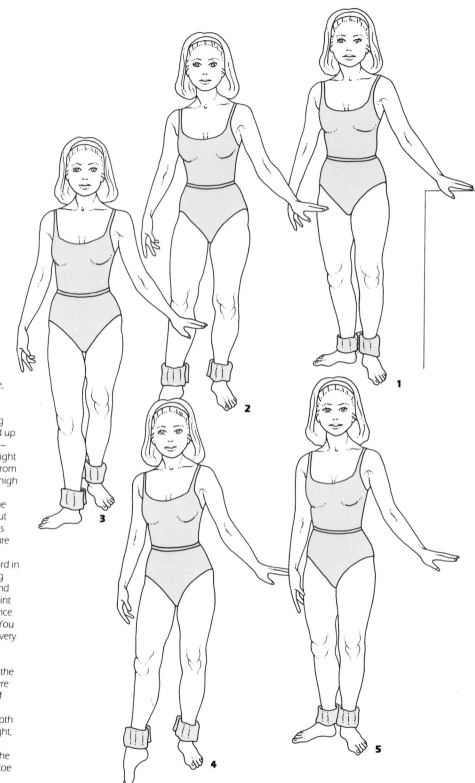

37 This is an adapted
ballet barre exercise,
which is marvelous for the
whole leg and the buttocks.
Stand with your hand resting
lightly on a chair back. Stand up
very tall with a straight back –
correct any arching with a slight
pelvic tilt. Turn out the legs from
the hip sockets, so that the thigh
and the butt muscles are
working, the knees above the
feet, **1**. Don't turn the feet out
further than the knees, as this
will throw your whole posture
out of alignment.

Take your right foot forward in
a straight line, really reaching
out of the hip socket to extend
the leg as far as it will go. Point
the foot and keep your balance
by lifting in the stomach, **2**. You
should feel the effect of this very
strongly in the thigh and the
buttock.

Keeping the turn-out, put the
heel on the floor. It is vital here
not to throw your hips out of
alignment or your weight
forward, though of course both
legs will be taking your weight,
3.

Now lift the heel, so that the
foot is pointed with just the toe

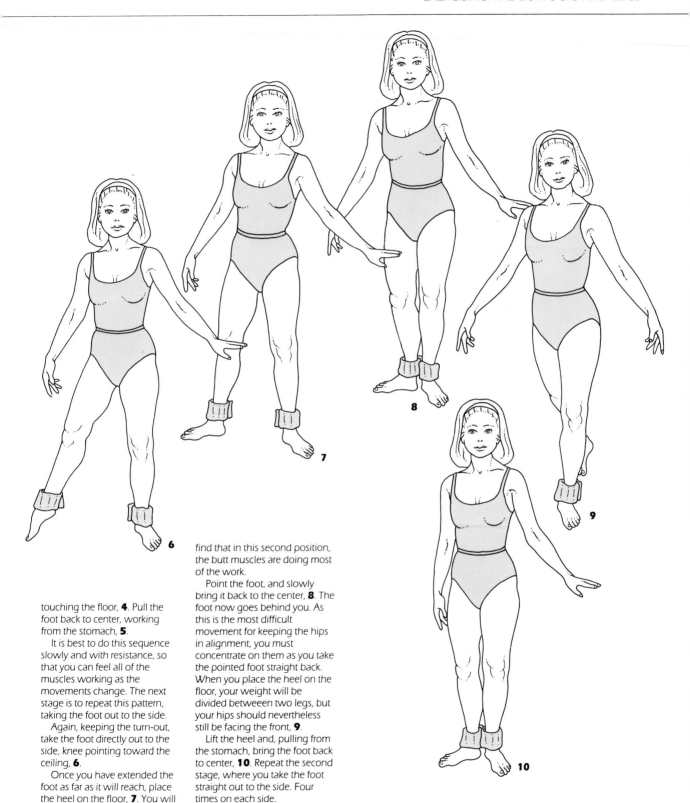

touching the floor, **4**. Pull the foot back to center, working from the stomach, **5**.

It is best to do this sequence slowly and with resistance, so that you can feel all of the muscles working as the movements change. The next stage is to repeat this pattern, taking the foot out to the side.

Again, keeping the turn-out, take the foot directly out to the side, knee pointing toward the ceiling, **6**.

Once you have extended the foot as far as it will reach, place the heel on the floor, **7**. You will find that in this second position, the butt muscles are doing most of the work.

Point the foot, and slowly bring it back to the center, **8**. The foot now goes behind you. As this is the most difficult movement for keeping the hips in alignment, you must concentrate on them as you take the pointed foot straight back. When you place the heel on the floor, your weight will be divided betweeen two legs, but your hips should nevertheless still be facing the front, **9**.

Lift the heel and, pulling from the stomach, bring the foot back to center, **10**. Repeat the second stage, where you take the foot straight out to the side. Four times on each side.

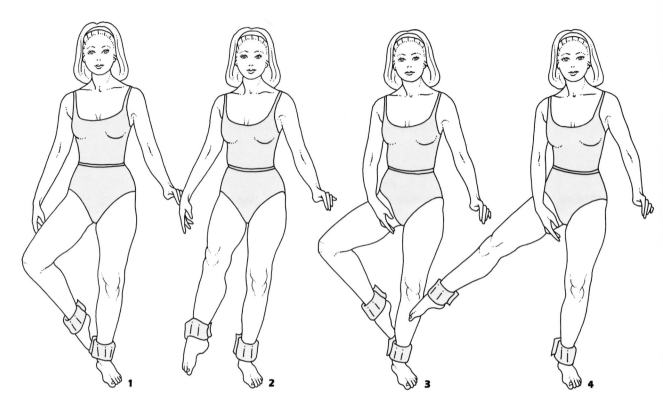

38 This exercise is another one based on ballet technique, following the pattern called "en croix" (in the shape of a cross). Again, you will need to pull up in the stomach for balance and, even more than in last exercise, to concentrate on not throwing your hips out of alignment as you lift the leg off the floor. Stand very tall, feet slightly turned out, left hand resting on a chair back. Lift the right leg, so that the toe is against the left ankle and the knee is pointing out to the side,**1**.

With a strongly pointed foot, stab the foot forward, so that it is still off the ground by a few inches, **2**. In ballet this movement is called frappé, "to strike or hit," and this describes prefectly the strength and suddenness for which you should be aiming.

Draw the foot back in toward you, so that the toe is again next to the ankle of the left leg,**3**. You should be able to feel the thigh muscles working hard to sustain the lift.

Using the same movement, take the foot out to the side, keeping the knee pointing to the ceiling,**4**. Lift up well in the body and in the stomach muscles, or you will find yourself leaning into the chair.

Draw the foot back in and now take it to the back,**5,6**. Don't try to get it too high, or your hips will be thrown out of line. Draw the foot back to the center, tucking your butt in as you do so, **7**.

Repeat the frappé to the side, **8**. Then repeat the sequence four times on each side.

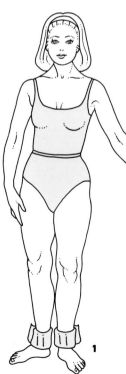

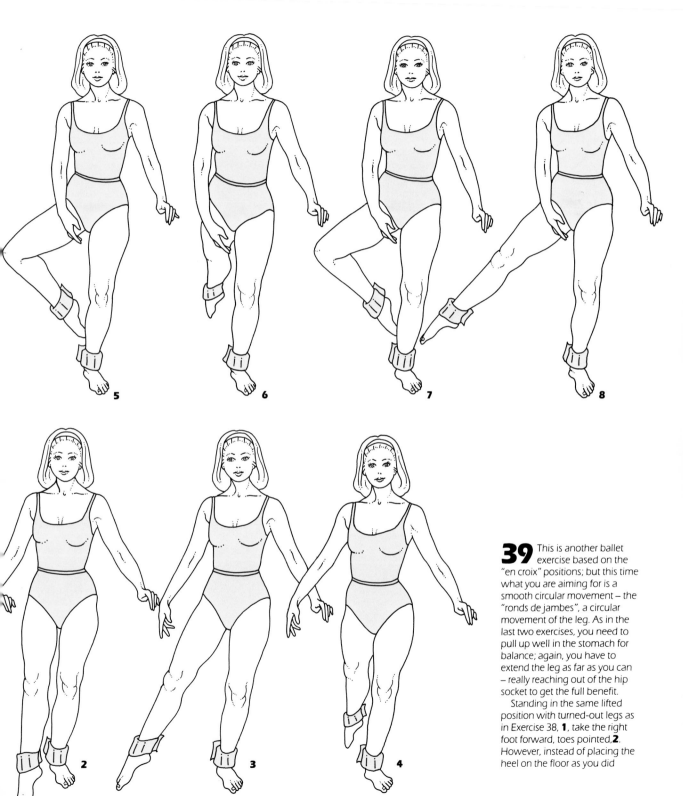

39 This is another ballet exercise based on the "en croix" positions; but this time what you are aiming for is a smooth circular movement – the "ronds de jambes", a circular movement of the leg. As in the last two exercises, you need to pull up well in the stomach for balance; again, you have to extend the leg as far as you can – really reaching out of the hip socket to get the full benefit.

Standing in the same lifted position with turned-out legs as in Exercise 38, **1**, take the right foot forward, toes pointed,**2**. However, instead of placing the heel on the floor as you did

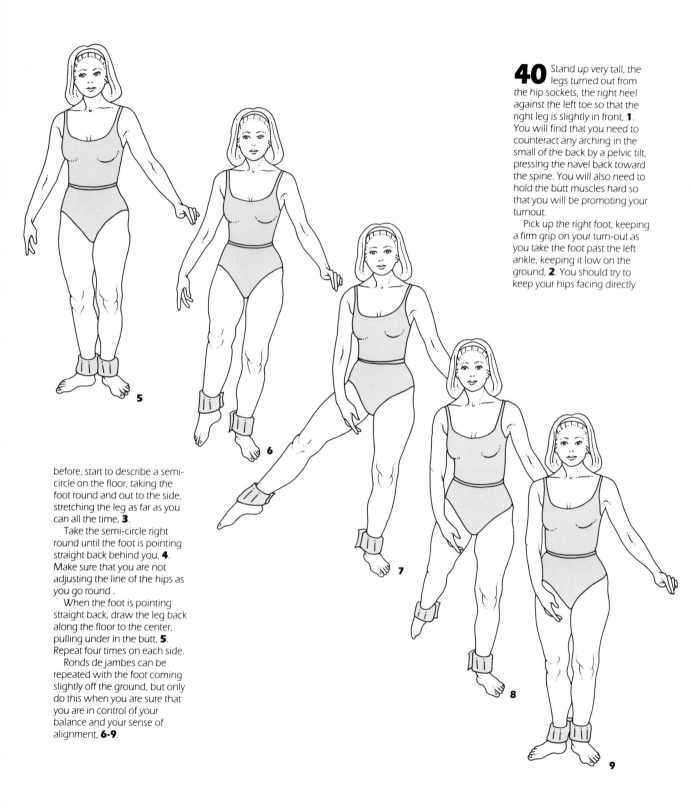

40 Stand up very tall, the legs turned out from the hip sockets, the right heel against the left toe so that the right leg is slightly in front, **1**. You will find that you need to counteract any arching in the small of the back by a pelvic tilt, pressing the navel back toward the spine. You will also need to hold the butt muscles hard so that you will be promoting your turnout.

Pick up the right foot, keeping a firm grip on your turn-out as you take the foot past the left ankle, keeping it low on the ground, **2**. You should try to keep your hips facing directly

before, start to describe a semi-circle on the floor, taking the foot round and out to the side, stretching the leg as far as you can all the time, **3**.

Take the semi-circle right round until the foot is pointing straight back behind you, **4**. Make sure that you are not adjusting the line of the hips as you go round.

When the foot is pointing straight back, draw the leg back along the floor to the center, pulling under in the butt, **5**. Repeat four times on each side.

Ronds de jambes can be repeated with the foot coming slightly off the ground, but only do this when you are sure that you are in control of your balance and your sense of alignment, **6-9**.

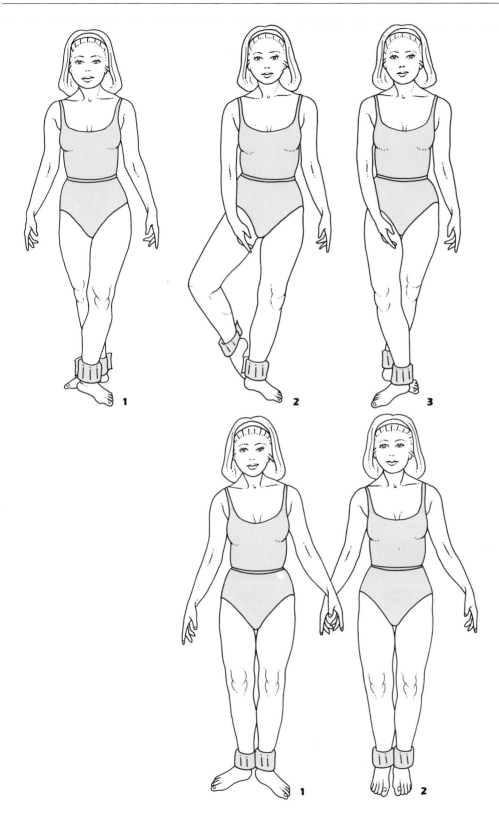

forward through this movement – don't allow yourself to wobble about too much. You will find that holding the stomach muscles firmly will help. As the foot is parallel with the ankle bone, the knee should be straight out at right-angles.

Put the left toe down behind the right heel and keeping your turn-out, put the rest of the foot on the floor, so that your feet are making the same pattern on the floor as they did to start with but are now reversed, **3.** You should feel a really strong stretch throughout the whole hip and thigh area. Providing you keep your turn-out at all times, this is one of the best exercises for toning up thighs and buttocks. Take the right foot back to the front passing through the same position as before. Eight on the right, then repeat on the left.

41 Stand up very tall, the upper body relaxed and any over-arching in the small of the back corrected with a pelvic tilt. Have the legs turned out, the knees directly over the feet, **1**. Now, very slowly, and without shifting your weight, draw the feet together, so that they are parallel, **2**. You will find this really works the inner thigh muscles.

Now reverse the action. Turn the legs out by really working the butt muscles and the thighs. You will find that, unless you have a strong hold on the stomach muscles, you may arch the back or throw yourself off balance. This is another marvelous exercise for the thighs and the buttocks. 16 complete movements.

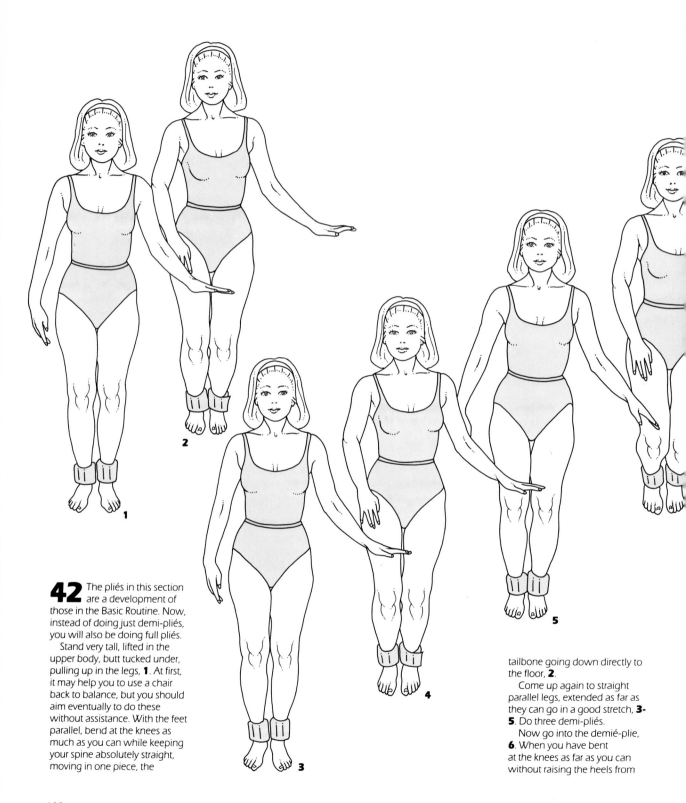

42 The pliés in this section are a development of those in the Basic Routine. Now, instead of doing just demi-pliés, you will also be doing full pliés.

Stand very tall, lifted in the upper body, butt tucked under, pulling up in the legs, **1**. At first, it may help you to use a chair back to balance, but you should aim eventually to do these without assistance. With the feet parallel, bend at the knees as much as you can while keeping your spine absolutely straight, moving in one piece, the

tailbone going down directly to the floor, **2**.

Come up again to straight parallel legs, extended as far as they can go in a good stretch, **3-5**. Do three demi-pliés.

Now go into the demié-plie, **6**. When you have bent at the knees as far as you can without raising the heels from

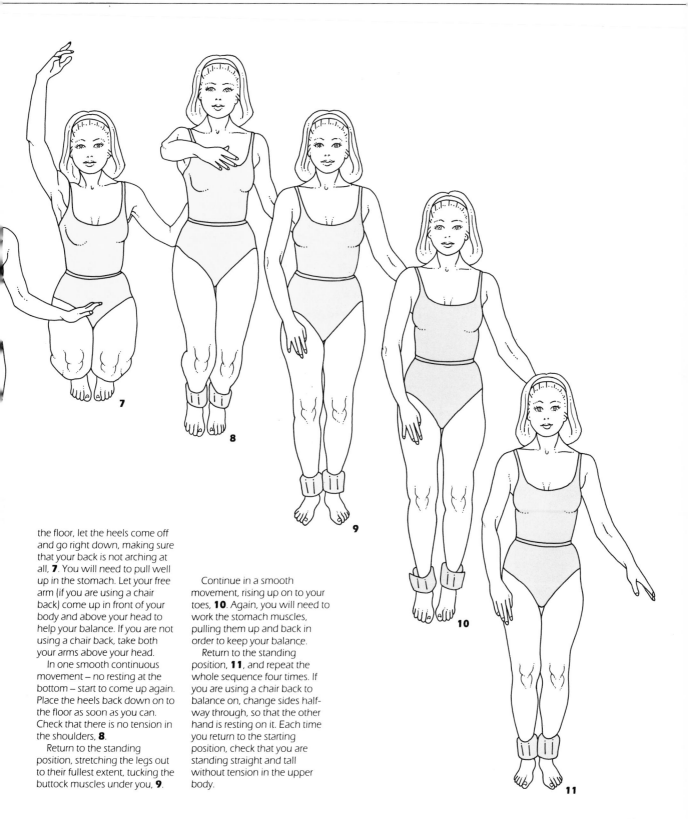

the floor, let the heels come off and go right down, making sure that your back is not arching at all, **7**. You will need to pull well up in the stomach. Let your free arm (if you are using a chair back) come up in front of your body and above your head to help your balance. If you are not using a chair back, take both your arms above your head.

In one smooth continuous movement – no resting at the bottom – start to come up again. Place the heels back down on to the floor as soon as you can. Check that there is no tension in the shoulders, **8**.

Return to the standing position, stretching the legs out to their fullest extent, tucking the buttock muscles under you, **9**.

Continue in a smooth movement, rising up on to your toes, **10**. Again, you will need to work the stomach muscles, pulling them up and back in order to keep your balance.

Return to the standing position, **11**, and repeat the whole sequence four times. If you are using a chair back to balance on, change sides half-way through, so that the other hand is resting on it. Each time you return to the starting position, check that you are standing straight and tall without tension in the upper body.

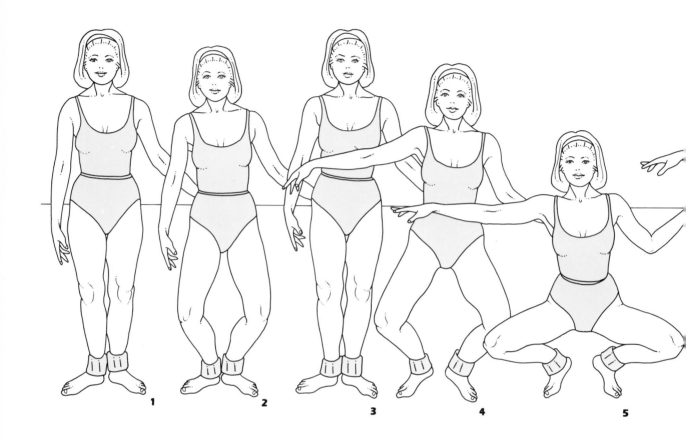

1　　2　　3　　4　　5

43 The second of the pliés is taken in first position, with the legs turning out from the hip sockets, knees above the feet, **1**. Really try to open out the pelvic area by tucking under the butt and wrapping round the inner thigh muscles – it's as if you were trying to get the inner thigh facing the front! If you are doing this properly and you are pulling up in the stomach, your back will always stay straight.

Bending at the knees and keeping the back straight, drop the tailbone down toward the floor as low as you can without taking your heels off the ground for three demi-pliés, **2**.

Return to the standing position, checking that you have

not thrown yourself off balance and that there is no tension in the shoulders or neck, **3**.

Now start to drop down again in the demi-plié as far as you can, **4**. Then allow your heels to come off and drop right down to the floor, **5**.

Make sure that you are still working the thigh and butt muscles hard, as well as pulling up in the stomach for balance. You can take your free arm out to the side for extra help with balance as you drop down. If you are not using a chair back for balance, take both arms out, but without tensing the shoulders or neck.

Don't rest at the bottom. As soon as you have reached down

as far as you can, start to rise up again, putting the heels down as quickly as possible, **6**.

Come back to the central standing position, extending the legs fully, **7**. Again, don't stop here – let the movement flow on and start to rise up on to your toes, **8**. You will find it much easier if you continue to squeeze your inner thighs together as you did when coming out of the plié.

Return to the starting position, **9**. Repeat the sequence four times, changing sides as before if you are using a chair back to aid your balance.

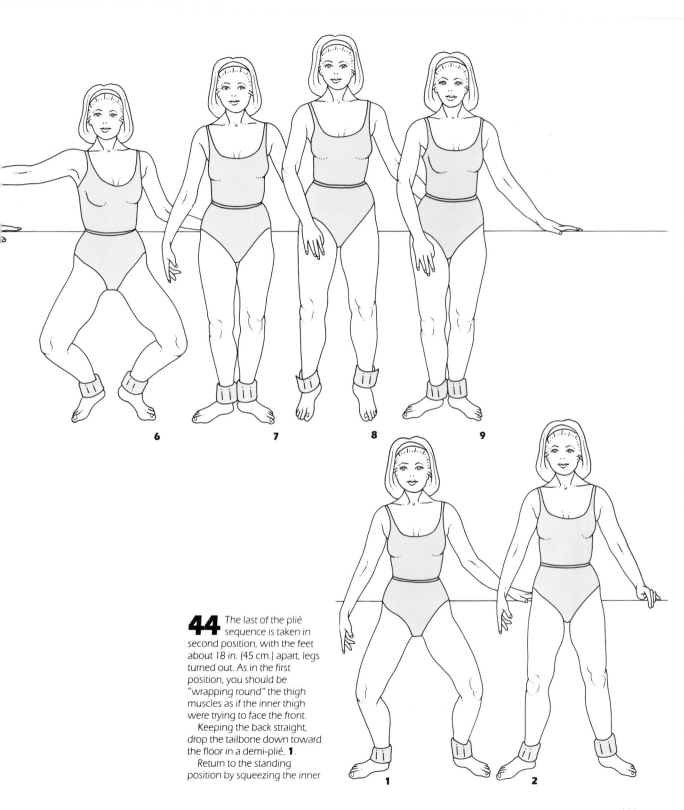

6　　　　**7**　　　　**8**　　　　**9**

44 The last of the plié sequence is taken in second position, with the feet about 18 in. (45 cm.) apart, legs turned out. As in the first position, you should be "wrapping round" the thigh muscles as if the inner thigh were trying to face the front.

Keeping the back straight, drop the tailbone down toward the floor in a demi-plié, **1**.

Return to the standing position by squeezing the inner

1　　　　**2**

thighs together and pulling in the butt and back thigh muscles, **2**. Repeat three times.

Start the demi-plié again. Keep your heels on the ground throughout, but drop down between the legs as far as you can, **3, 4, 5**.

Rise up through the center, squeezing the inner thighs together, passing through the standing position, **6**. Continue in one smooth movement, rising up on to your toes, **7**. Return to the standing position, still keeping your turn-out and tucking your butt well under. Repeat four times right through, changing sides if you are using a chair back.

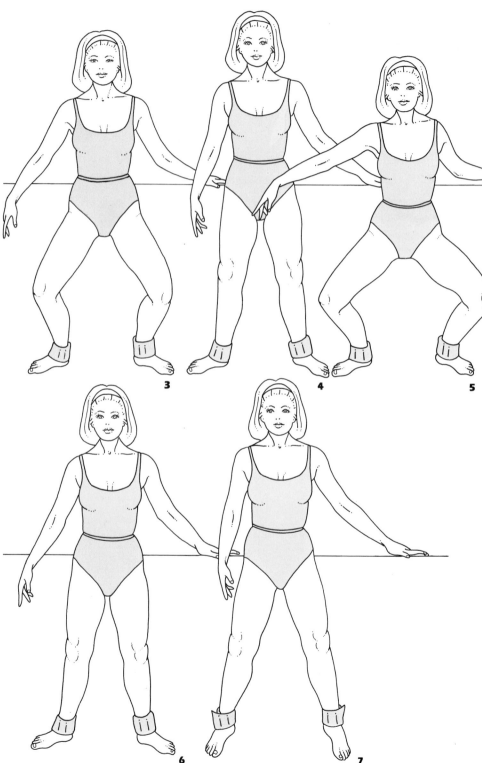

3

4

5

6

7

45 Stand up very tall, legs turned out from the hip sockets, pulling the tailbone down and "wrapping round" the thigh muscles to emphasize the turn-out, **1**. Your feet will make a V-shape on the floor; as always, make sure that the knees are directly above them and not rolling inward. Now pick up the right leg, bending at the knee, and turn it in so that it comes across the front of the body, **2**. You can help your balance by resting your left hand on the back of a chair.

Now turn the leg out from the hip socket so that your right knee is pointing straight out to the side, the right ankle crossing in front of the left knee, **3**.

Take the right knee as high as you can without losing the turn-out – this will mean working the butt and thigh muscles very hard, **4**. Keeping the butt tucked under will also help with your balance.

Now turn the leg from the hip socket, so that you start to turn in to cross the right leg in front of your body again. This is a figure-eight movement which you trace with your knee, and is another excellent exercise for the thighs, **5, 6**. Eight figure-eights on each side.

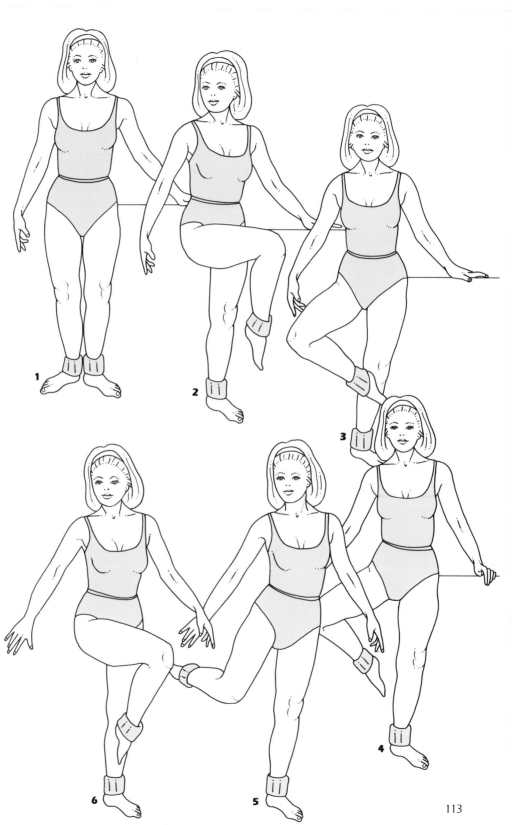

113

46 This exercise will tone up your inner thigh muscles. Lie on your side, the upper body propped up on one elbow, the other hand in front of the body for balance. Put your top leg on a chair, the knee facing forward. Make sure that you are not arching your back – your spine should be quite straight. The legs should be fully extended and pulling away from the body, **1**.

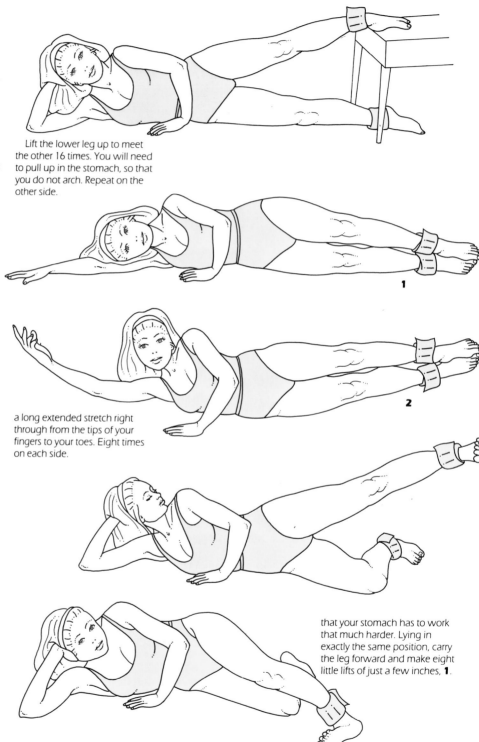

Lift the lower leg up to meet the other 16 times. You will need to pull up in the stomach, so that you do not arch. Repeat on the other side.

47 This exercise is a harder variation of the last one – it works the stomach very hard indeed! Lie flat on the floor, the lower arm extended above the head, **1**. The line from your extended hand through the spine to your pointed feet should be absolutely straight.

Using the upper arm on the floor in front of you for balance, pull up hard in the stomach and raise the legs, upper body and arm, so that you make a long low curve, **2**. This does not mean, though, that the body hunches up in any way – this is

a long extended stretch right through from the tips of your fingers to your toes. Eight times on each side.

48 Lie on the floor with your lower leg bent at the knee, the upper body propped up on the elbow. Again, making sure that your back is completely straight and pressing your navel toward your spine, raise the top leg, extending it as far as possible away from you and flexing the foot, **1**. Keeping the leg quite straight, make 16 little circles in this lifted position, first clockwise, then counter clockwise, on both legs.

49 This exercise is very similar to the last one, but this time you take the leg forward, so that it is at right angles to your body. This means

that your stomach has to work that much harder. Lying in exactly the same position, carry the leg forward and make eight little lifts of just a few inches, **1**.

50 This exercise and the following ones use double weights. Lie on your side, the lower leg bent at the knee, the lower arm stretched out above your head. Use the top arm to secure your balance by resting the hand on the floor. Have one weight on the ankle of the upper leg and put the other one around the foot. Stretching right out of the hip with the upper leg, the foot flexed back hard and the heel

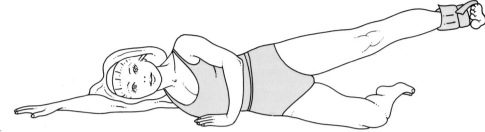

leading the way, make eight long, slow lifts, feeling the stretch right down the body and out through the leg, **1**. Repeat on the other side.

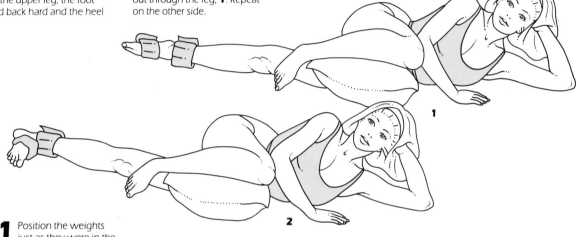

51 Position the weights just as they were in the last exercise, but this time on the lower leg. Lie on your side, propped up on one elbow. Bend the top leg and rest the knee on a cushion or pillow, so that the whole leg is lifted from the floor, **1**. Flex the foot of the lower leg and, extending the leg as far as you can in a straight line away from the body, make eight little lifts, **2**. Repeat on the other side. Do both of these last execises with your back against a wall to check that you are keeping absolutely straight.

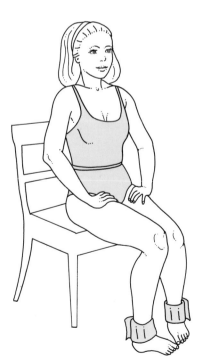

52 This is a wonderful exercise for trimming the ankles and calves. Sit on the edge of a chair, feet flat on the floor, hands resting on your thighs, upper body relaxed. Keep your knees together, but take the heels out, so that they are about six inches apart, but still on the floor. Keep the toes together.

Sweep the toes out and upward, so that they make a little semi-circle and come off the floor, **1**. The knees remain together throughout . Sweep out and in 16 times. This is a very strong movement indeed!

SUPPLENESS

The exercises in this section use a lot of stretching and so they should only be done after your body is completely warmed up. You will find that you are naturally more supple then and can take the stretches further. Several of the exercises here are based on dance movements and not only stretch and open up the body but aim to give fluidity and lightness of movement.

Everyone has areas of tightness – often one side of the body is visibly more loose than the other. You will become aware of this as you exercise and you can then concentrate on the problem areas accordingly . You will find that regular, gentle stretching will open up any stiff areas far more effectively than trying to force yourself into difficult positions – so give yourself time.

The one area to take special care of in these suppleness exercises is the back. If your back is not strong or you have any problems with it, don't do any of the exercises where it needs to arch. And, as always, keep the navel pressed well back toward the spine.

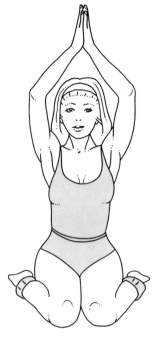

55 This exercise stretches out the front of the legs. It is very tough, so don't do it if you feel any pain in your knees. Sit kneeling between your legs – ideally you should actually be sitting on the floor between your legs. If you find this difficult, sit on a cushion, so that you don't have to drop down so far.

Take your arms above your head, palms together, elbows wide open, **1**. Keeping the shoulders pulled down, raise the hands. Do eight little lifts, unless you feel a lot of tension coming into the neck. In such a case, drop the arms down straight away and roll the shoulders in a circular movement to release them.

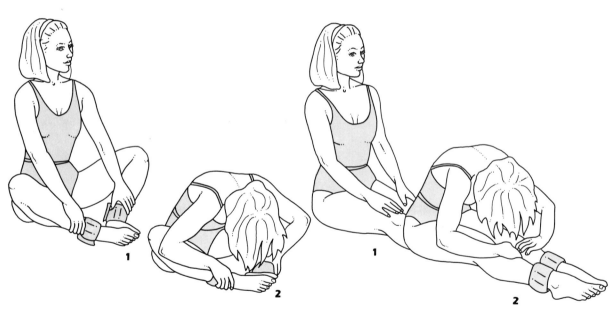

53 Sit up tall with the soles of your feet together, hands on the ankles, **1**. Curve in the back and roll forward; your head reaching down toward your feet, **2**. 16 stretches then roll up through the spine to a straight back.

54 Sit up straight with your legs parallel, out in front of you, with toes pointed, **1**.
Curving over in the back, reach down toward the ankles for 16 stretches, **2**. Eventually you should aim to get the body flat against the legs, but this will not be possible at the start.

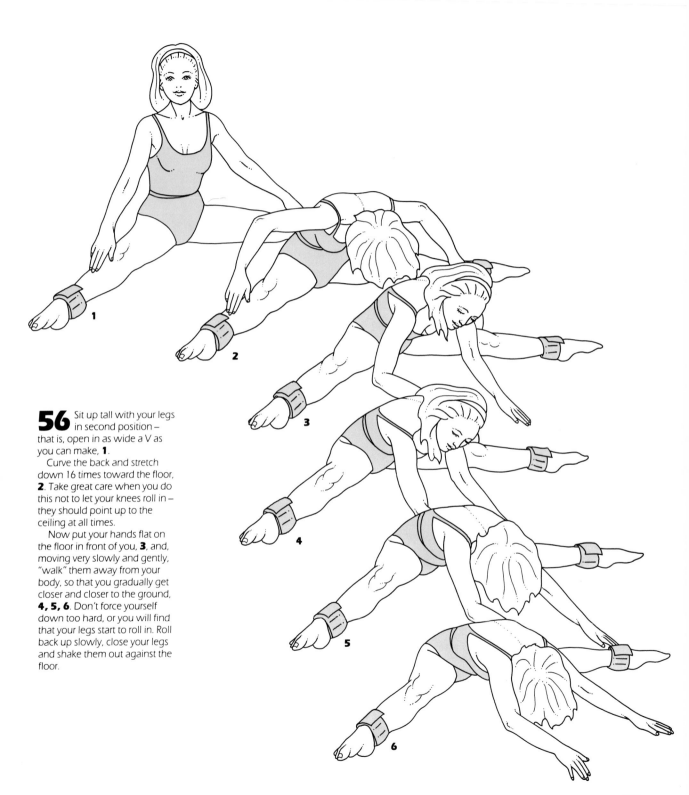

56 Sit up tall with your legs in second position – that is, open in as wide a V as you can make, **1**.

Curve the back and stretch down 16 times toward the floor, **2**. Take great care when you do this not to let your knees roll in – they should point up to the ceiling at all times.

Now put your hands flat on the floor in front of you, **3**, and, moving very slowly and gently, "walk" them away from your body, so that you gradually get closer and closer to the ground, **4, 5, 6**. Don't force yourself down too hard, or you will find that your legs start to roll in. Roll back up slowly, close your legs and shake them out against the floor.

57 This is a cat-like stretch; it should not be attempted if you have any weakness in the back. Your head should be in line with the rest of your spine, **1**.

Pull back in the stomach and arch up, dropping your head down. Iron out the back again so that it is completely flat, neck and head in line, **2**.

Now arch the other way so that you look up and curve in the small of the back, **3**. As this is the most strenuous part of the exercise, approach it with care. If you know that you have a weak back, leave this part out and just use the first arch, alternating with the flat back. Repeat the whole sequence four times.

58 This exercise follows on from the last and, again, should only be undertaken if your back is strong enough to do it without the risk of strain. Start in the same position as the last exercise, on all fours, spine in a long straight line, **1**.

Raise the right knee in to the chest, rounding the back and dropping the head down to meet the knee, **2**.

Then, straighten the leg, reaching it up and back. Curve the back so that you look up in a long stretch, **3**. Repeat the whole sequence eight times on each leg.

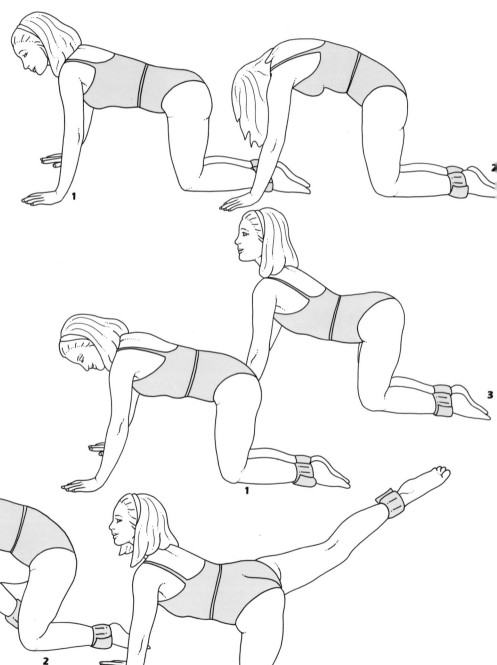

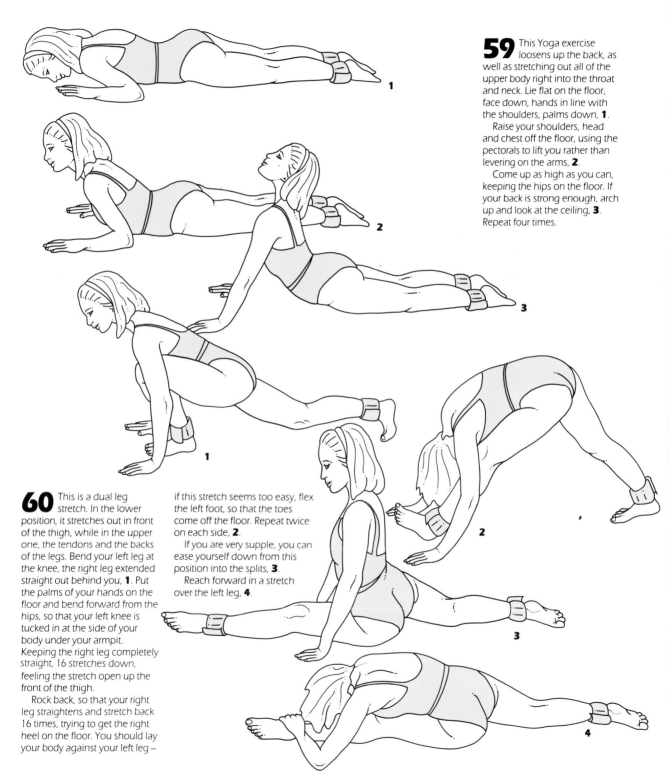

59 This Yoga exercise loosens up the back, as well as stretching out all of the upper body right into the throat and neck. Lie flat on the floor, face down, hands in line with the shoulders, palms down, **1**.

Raise your shoulders, head and chest off the floor, using the pectorals to lift you rather than levering on the arms, **2**.

Come up as high as you can, keeping the hips on the floor. If your back is strong enough, arch up and look at the ceiling, **3**. Repeat four times.

60 This is a dual leg stretch. In the lower position, it stretches out in front of the thigh, while in the upper one, the tendons and the backs of the legs. Bend your left leg at the knee, the right leg extended straight out behind you, **1**. Put the palms of your hands on the floor and bend forward from the hips, so that your left knee is tucked in at the side of your body under your armpit. Keeping the right leg completely straight, 16 stretches down, feeling the stretch open up the front of the thigh.

Rock back, so that your right leg straightens and stretch back 16 times, trying to get the right heel on the floor. You should lay your body against your left leg –

if this stretch seems too easy, flex the left foot, so that the toes come off the floor. Repeat twice on each side, **2**.

If you are very supple, you can ease yourself down from this position into the splits, **3**.

Reach forward in a stretch over the left leg, **4**.

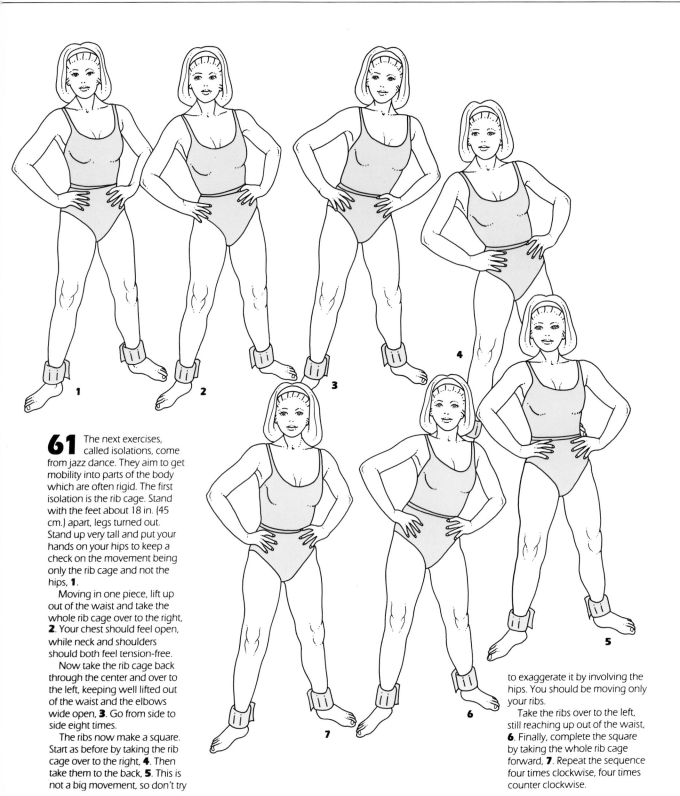

61 The next exercises, called isolations, come from jazz dance. They aim to get mobility into parts of the body which are often rigid. The first isolation is the rib cage. Stand with the feet about 18 in. (45 cm.) apart, legs turned out. Stand up very tall and put your hands on your hips to keep a check on the movement being only the rib cage and not the hips, **1**.

Moving in one piece, lift up out of the waist and take the whole rib cage over to the right, **2**. Your chest should feel open, while neck and shoulders should both feel tension-free.

Now take the rib cage back through the center and over to the left, keeping well lifted out of the waist and the elbows wide open, **3**. Go from side to side eight times.

The ribs now make a square. Start as before by taking the rib cage over to the right, **4**. Then take them to the back, **5**. This is not a big movement, so don't try

to exaggerate it by involving the hips. You should be moving only your ribs.

Take the ribs over to the left, still reaching up out of the waist, **6**. Finally, complete the square by taking the whole rib cage forward, **7**. Repeat the sequence four times clockwise, four times counter clockwise.

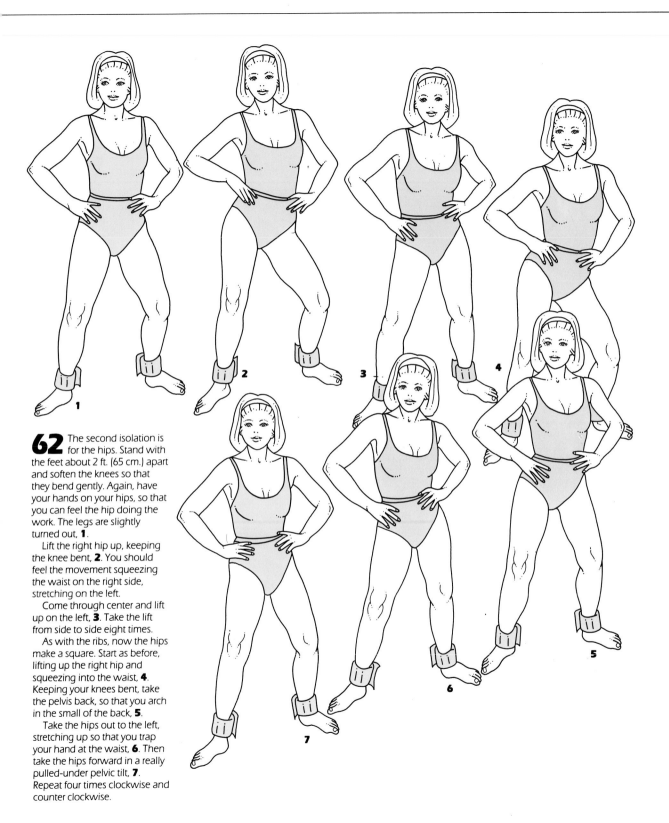

62 The second isolation is for the hips. Stand with the feet about 2 ft. (65 cm.) apart and soften the knees so that they bend gently. Again, have your hands on your hips, so that you can feel the hip doing the work. The legs are slightly turned out, **1**.

Lift the right hip up, keeping the knee bent, **2**. You should feel the movement squeezing the waist on the right side, stretching on the left.

Come through center and lift up on the left, **3**. Take the lift from side to side eight times.

As with the ribs, now the hips make a square. Start as before, lifting up the right hip and squeezing into the waist, **4**. Keeping your knees bent, take the pelvis back, so that you arch in the small of the back, **5**.

Take the hips out to the left, stretching up so that you trap your hand at the waist, **6**. Then take the hips forward in a really pulled-under pelvic tilt, **7**. Repeat four times clockwise and counter clockwise.

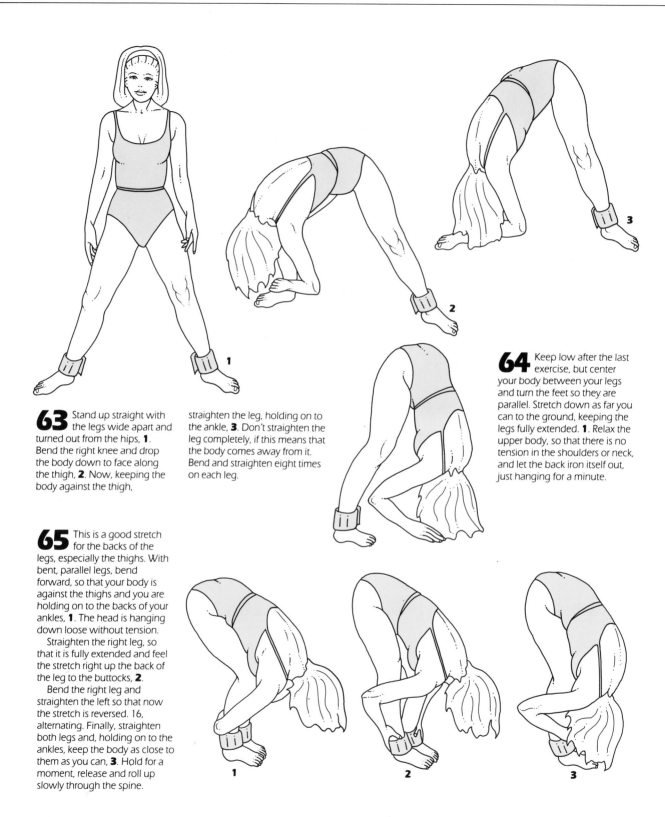

63 Stand up straight with the legs wide apart and turned out from the hips, **1**. Bend the right knee and drop the body down to face along the thigh, **2**. Now, keeping the body against the thigh, straighten the leg, holding on to the ankle, **3**. Don't straighten the leg completely, if this means that the body comes away from it. Bend and straighten eight times on each leg.

64 Keep low after the last exercise, but center your body between your legs and turn the feet so they are parallel. Stretch down as far you can to the ground, keeping the legs fully extended. **1**. Relax the upper body, so that there is no tension in the shoulders or neck, and let the back iron itself out, just hanging for a minute.

65 This is a good stretch for the backs of the legs, especially the thighs. With bent, parallel legs, bend forward, so that your body is against the thighs and you are holding on to the backs of your ankles, **1**. The head is hanging down loose without tension.

Straighten the right leg, so that it is fully extended and feel the stretch right up the back of the leg to the buttocks, **2**.

Bend the right leg and straighten the left so that now the stretch is reversed. 16, alternating. Finally, straighten both legs and, holding on to the ankles, keep the body as close to them as you can, **3**. Hold for a moment, release and roll up slowly through the spine.

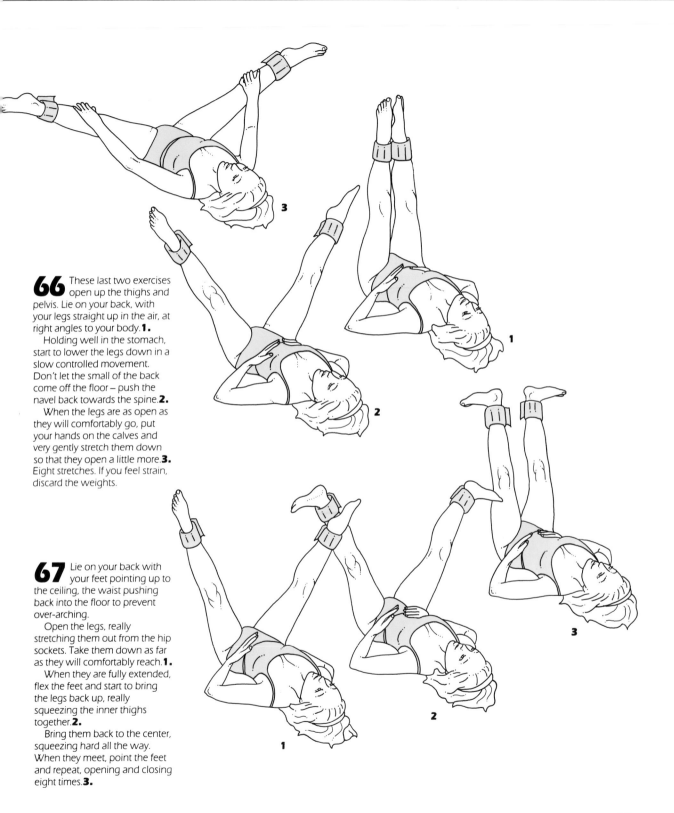

66 These last two exercises open up the thighs and pelvis. Lie on your back, with your legs straight up in the air, at right angles to your body.**1.**

Holding well in the stomach, start to lower the legs down in a slow controlled movement. Don't let the small of the back come off the floor – push the navel back towards the spine.**2.**

When the legs are as open as they will comfortably go, put your hands on the calves and very gently stretch them down so that they open a little more.**3.** Eight stretches. If you feel strain, discard the weights.

67 Lie on your back with your feet pointing up to the ceiling, the waist pushing back into the floor to prevent over-arching.

Open the legs, really stretching them out from the hip sockets. Take them down as far as they will comfortably reach.**1.**

When they are fully extended, flex the feet and start to bring the legs back up, really squeezing the inner thighs together.**2.**

Bring them back to the center, squeezing hard all the way. When they meet, point the feet and repeat, opening and closing eight times.**3.**

Stretching and Relaxing

By providing you with strength, suppleness and stamina, the exercises in this book will help you to create a well-toned body. However, since mind and body are inextricably linked, the following relaxation exercises are specifically designed to help you bring both together in a similarly well-tuned state.

The exercises follow on naturally from the breathings at the end of the cooling-down exercises at the end of the Basic Routine. They may also be used independently to dispel tension and stress – which contribute to many common ailments, such as headaches and indigestion – and may even help you cope with ulcers and heart disease. They may also relieve insomnia – they will improve the chances of sleep – and help, too, to counteract anxiety and depression.

How do relaxation exercises differ from just putting your feet up and having a rest? They differ because, through following this routine, you learn to relax consciously, one by one, all the muscles in your body and face (surprisingly enough, a storehouse of tension), while the deep breathings fill your body with revitalizing oxygen in a way which is very different from normal shallow breathing.

All in all, deep relaxation is a great restorative. In fact, in Yoga, where relaxation and breathing techniques are developed much further than they are here, it is taught that what we breathe in is prana, or the life force itself. This is a very useful image on which to concentrate when it comes to the breathings during relaxation.

Ten minutes of deep relaxation can be as refreshing as a good night's sleep. So try it when you are feeling at a low ebb, tired, nervously frazzled, or simply when you need to find your second wind.

STRETCHES

The stretches here should either follow the breathings as you finish the Basic Routine, or be preceded by a short warm-up – the first exercise in the Basic Routine, for instance. The weights are not used.

As you relax, your body temperature will drop, so you should wear more than you would while exercising conventionally, though what you choose should be loose and unconstricting. When it comes to the deep relaxation which follows these exercises, it can be a good idea to cover yourself with a blanket.

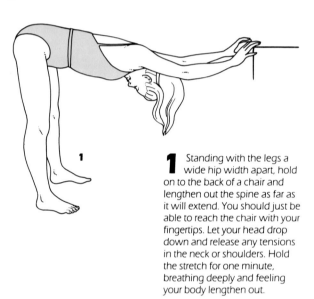

1 Standing with the legs a wide hip width apart, hold on to the back of a chair and lengthen out the spine as far as it will extend. You should just be able to reach the chair with your fingertips. Let your head drop down and release any tensions in the neck or shoulders. Hold the stretch for one minute, breathing deeply and feeling your body lengthen out.

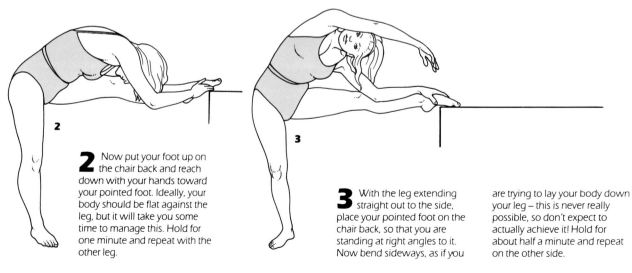

2 Now put your foot up on the chair back and reach down with your hands toward your pointed foot. Ideally, your body should be flat against the leg, but it will take you some time to manage this. Hold for one minute and repeat with the other leg.

3 With the leg extending straight out to the side, place your pointed foot on the chair back, so that you are standing at right angles to it. Now bend sideways, as if you are trying to lay your body down your leg – this is never really possible, so don't expect to actually achieve it! Hold for about half a minute and repeat on the other side.

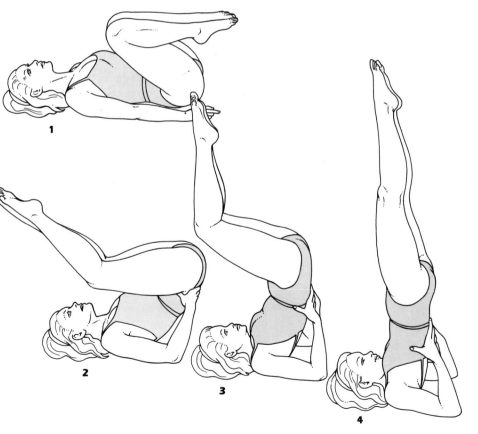

4 Now lie down on the floor, your arms stretched out straight from the shoulders. Bend your knees up to the ceiling and, as you drop them out to the side, turn your head to face the opposite direction. You should feel a strong diagonal stretch right through the body.

5 Bring the knees up to the center at the same time as you move your head back, so you are looking at the ceiling.

6 Now drop the knees down the other side, turning your face away from them. Alternate four times on each side. To make sure that you are keeping your knees firmly together, you can put a tennis ball between them.

Now lie down and lengthen your spine along the floor, so that you iron out any bumps in it, and try to flatten the small of your back into the floor. If you find this uncomfortable, or feel that your back is over-arching, bend your knees up over a chair. Otherwise your legs should be straight down from the hips, rolling out slightly in a relaxed position. Feel your neck as a continuation of your spine, stretched out fully and in line. You will find this means that your chin tilts down toward your chest. Your arms should be relaxed at the sides of your body.

THE SHOULDER STAND

1 Lying flat on the floor, breathe in and bend your knees in to your chest, feeling the neck lengthen.

2 As you breathe out, begin to raise your back from the floor, supporting your hips with your hands. Your feet will be pointing back over your head.

3 Start to straighten out your spine until you reach a vertical position. This needs a fair amount of practice.

4 With the legs raised up straight in line and the feet pointed, press your chin to your chest. This stimulates the thyroid and parathyroid glands, which have been called the youth glands because they supposedly delay signs of aging. Close your eyes, breathe deeply and try to relax. At first, you will be able to hold this pose and the following one for only a short time. Try, though, to hold them for longer as you get used to the positions.

THE PLOUGH

1 Lying flat on the floor, bend your knees in to your chest as you did for the shoulder stand.

2 Supporting your hips as you did before, start to raise the lower back up from the floor until the feet are pointing back over the head.

3 Instead of rolling up through the spine so that your legs are vertical, take your legs horizontally behind your head when you roll up. Your legs and spine should be straight.

When you can do this pose comfortably, you can flex the feet back, so that they are "on the walk", toes curled under. Come out of both of these poses by dropping your knees down to your chest, rolling through the spine and then stretching your legs out along the floor.

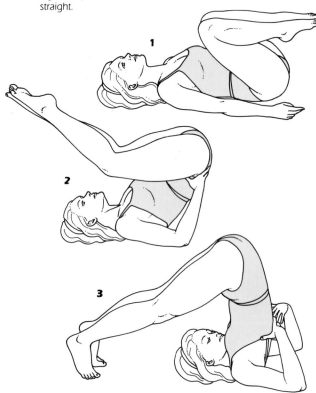

THE SLOPE

If you don't feel up to these yoga poses, you can still benefit by assuming any slightly inverted position. For this, you will need a firm plank, with one end securely raised at least a foot from the ground. Lie down on this with your feet at the top, your head at the bottom.

THE RELAXATION SEQUENCE

During relaxation, your body temperature will drop, so now is the time to cover yourself with a blanket, or to put on an extra layer of clothing.

Before you can relax your muscles, you need to be aware of them. So the sequence starts at the feet and works its way up, the aim being to establish a rhythm of tensing and relaxing.

1 Lie down on the floor as described at the end of the stretches earlier in this section. Don't lie on a bed, as it will be too soft, and choose as quiet and as airy a room as possible. The routine may take you only 10 minutes, but these are precious; you will not want to be disturbed, so take the 'phone off the hook.

2 Close your eyes and give yourself a few moments in which to become aware of the weight of your whole body, softening and spreading out on the floor after the exertions of exercise and stretching. Check that there is no tension in the neck by rolling the head from side to side.

3 Stretch your feet and legs out from the hip sockets. Hold the tension for a few seconds and then let it go and relax, feeling feet and legs rolling out gently. Clench your buttocks and relax them. Let your back lengthen and straighten against the floor.

4 Squeeze your vaginal and abdominal muscles and then let them go. Feel any tension in the neck and shoulders drop away, elongate the neck, so that there is no hunching in the shoulder area, but lots of space, and then stretch out the arms, letting them roll out to the sides. Make a fist with each hand in turn, stretch the fingers, then let them soften into a relaxed position.

Squeeze all of the facial muscles and then let them go. Feel your forehead relax and any tension or frowning soften away. Let the lower jaw slacken, so that your teeth are not clenched together, your tongue should not cleave to the roof of your mouth, but spread out behind your bottom teeth. Let your eyes roll back behind the lids and the muscles around the eyes relax.

Your whole body should now feel heavy, limp and lifeless. Concentrate now on your breathing, feeling the oxygen coming in to your lungs filling them with air and then expelling the used stale air. Feel each breath recharging your physical and mental batteries and slowing down the tempo of your whole body. Try to deepen the breathing, so that the air fills not just your lungs but your abdomen which should rise as you inhale. Gradually return to normal, regulated breathing, feeling the air's revitalizing and relaxing effects.

Remain in this state of deep relaxation for at least five minutes and then come back slowly. Begin by taking a few deep breaths and, if you feel like it, stretch and yawn. Roll over on to your side before you sit up.

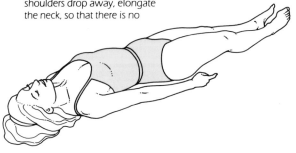

SALUTE TO THE SUN

This is one of the best known yoga asanas and will stimulate your whole body.

Stand very tall, butt tucked under, stomach lifted, the arms bent at the elbows and the hands together in a prayer position. Breathe in deeply and then exhale.

1 Now breathe in deeply and stretch the arms back over the head, curving the back at the same time.

2 As you breathe out, bend from the hips with a straight back. Aim to get your hands on the floor or holding the backs of your ankles, but don't force this.

3 Breathe in and take your right leg out behind you, stretching it fully. The body is in line with the bent left leg and you arch your back to look up.

4 Take your left leg back so that it is in line with the right and you are supported on your arms. Legs and spine should make a triangle. Breathe out.

5 Supporting your weight on your hands, drop your knees and chest to the ground – your hips are still lifted, though.

6 As you breathe in, drop the hips to the floor and bend back to look up, the whole spine arching from the hips.

7 As you breathe out, return to the triangle shape, really stretching out and trying to press your heels into the floor.

8 Breathe in and stretch your left leg out behind you, arching back to look up.

9 Breathe out as you bring the left leg back in line with the right and, keeping the back straight, bend forward, trying to press the body against the legs. Again, if necessary, bend the knees.

10 Breathe in, raising the body from the hips and bending with an arched back and arms outstretched.

11 Breathe out and return to the starting position.

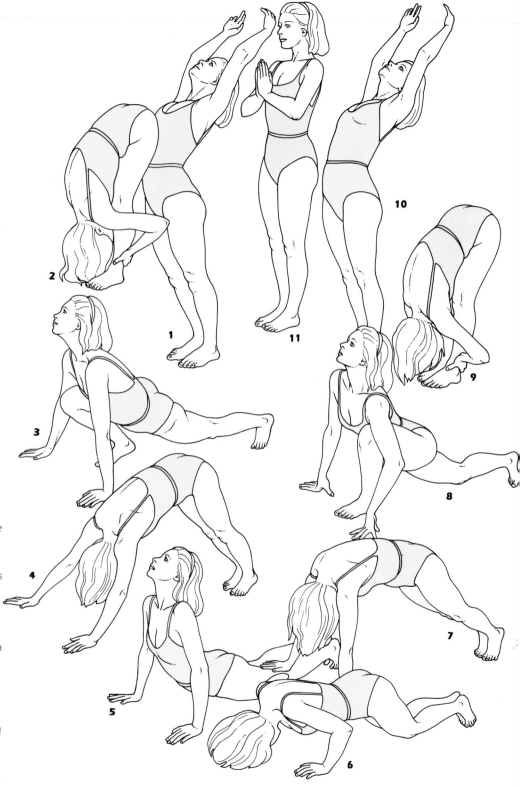